How To Have A Girl

A Step-By-Step Guide to Scientifically Maximize Your Chances of Conceiving a Daughter

By

J. Martin Young, M.D., F.A.A.P.

1st Edition

A Young Idea!

Young Ideas
Publishing Division
Amarillo, Texas

How To Have A Girl

A Step-By-Step Guide to Scientfically Maximize Your Chances of Conceiving a Daughter
By J. Martin Young, M.D., F.A.A.P.

Young Ideas
Publishing Division
1600 S. Coulter, Bldg. C, Suite 304
Amarillo, Texas 79106

Copyright © 1995
First Printing 1995
Printed in the United States of America

Library of Congress Catalog Card Number: 94-61630
Young, M.D., J. Martin
How To Have A Girl: A Step-By-Step Guide to Scientifically Maximize Your Chances of
Conceiving a Daughter / by J. Martin Young, M.D. — 1st edition.

ISBN 0-9643420-2-2: $19.95 Softcover

Cover Photography: Steve Satterwhite Photography, Amarillo, Texas

Cover Design: Dana Bottlinger, Young Ideas Publishing Division, Amarillo, Texas

Cover Layout: Trafton Printing, Amarillo, Texas

Printed by BookCrafters, Chelsea, Michigan, USA

PREFACE

Sex preselection is the attempt to choose or influence the sex of an unborn child, and couples have attempted sex preselection throughout recorded history. However, during the first half of this century, techniques were not widely practiced. Families were large, and it was rare for one sex to not be represented. Unfortunately, children are now an economic liability often requiring support into their early twenties, and the number of children in American families has steadily fallen. In particular, professional couples, with expanding time requirements, are often choosing to conceive only one or two children. Since couples having random intercourse will have only a 50% chance of conceiving either a boy or a girl, only half of the couples who have two children will have a child of each sex. Boys and girls are socialized differently in America, and, unfortunately, couples with all boys or all girls will miss out on one of these experiences.

I was not interested in sex preselection until after numerous families in my practice asked me for advice on how to influence the sex of their next child. I initially discussed the subject with friends and relatives who gave me a copy of the book, *Your Baby's Sex: now you can choose*, written by Dr. Landrum B. Shettles and David Rorvik. I was very excited until I inspected the front cover and found the publication date of 1970, over 20 years earlier. The next day, I visited the library and used their computers to search the Medline computer data bases of the National Library of Medicine. To my surprise, I found numerous research articles concerning the factors which influence the sex of children, and the most recent articles consistently refuted the recommendations of Dr. Shettles' book.

It took only a few weeks to formulate methods which would allow average couples to increase their chances of either a boy or a girl. This information initially took the form of a brief outline, but, as the number of requests steadily increased, it grew into two separate books: *How To Have A Boy* and *How To Have A Girl*. Since that time, numerous couples have used my methods and made helpful suggestions. I cannot guarantee that you will conceive a female child, but the methods in this book can increase your chances to well above that of the general population, in your own home without the use of drugs or special procedures.

"Read not to contradict and confute; nor to believe and take for granted; nor to find talk and discourse; but to weigh and consider." **Francis Bacon**

FOREWORD

J. Martin Young is an outstanding physician. Having learned medicine with him, I can attest to his intelligence and diligence in his search for the truth. A quick review of his bibliography and of Chapter 3, particularly Figure 3-1, will attest to the length to which he has gone to research the facts. Fortunately, he has also gone to great lengths to present them in a very readable fashion to people with little or no background knowledge.

When he first told me of his plan to write such a book, I was pessimistic. I was not aware of any verifiable data which showed anyone could do anything to alter the male:female ratio of zygotes (fertilized eggs) beyond 50:50. Obviously, I was not fully informed. To quote Dr. Joycelyn Elders, "I hadn't educated 'me' yet." Dr. Young has sighted study after study showing just that. No one can guarantee a boy or a girl, but the information presented here can increase your chances of having a girl to significantly higher than the average couple..

I need to warn you. Dr. Young is fairly compulsive, and he asks you to be fairly compulsive in tracking the menstrual cycle in order to maximize the odds of having a girl. However, he does provide detailed flowcharts which will greatly assist you in keeping the records needed. I think you will find this book to be a valuable resource. Enjoy it!

James "Whit" Walker, M.D.

Dedication

This book is dedicated to my wife, Dana. The only thing that takes more dedication than performing home sex preselection is tolerating your husband while he writes a book on the subject. It is also dedicated to my three beautiful daughters: Caitlyn, Christian, and Callan. If I had only known then ...

"The road to success is filled with women pushing their husbands along."
Lord Dewar

Acknowledgements

Peer Review:
    James "Whit" Walker, Jr., M.D., A.C.I.M.
    C. Edward Sauer, Jr., D.D.S.
    Henry Robinson, P.A.
    Jerrod Roberts, R.Ph.

Style Review:
    T. David Cullar
    Stephen and Samia Zolnerowich
    Kip (Mr. Enthusiasm) and Dawn Fuller

"No matter what accomplishments you achieve, somebody helps you."
Aletha Gibson

Finally, I want to thank Jack and Joyce Young -- my parents and my friends:
"The mark of a true champion is to come from behind and win."
Unknown

About the Author........

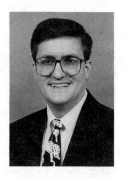

Dr. Young has a large solo private pediatric practice in Amarillo, Texas. He received his undergraduate education at Midwestern State University graduating summa cum laude as the highest ranking graduate in consecutive years: 1985 with a B.S. in Chemistry and 1986 with a B.S. in both Biology and Psychology. He attended medical school at the University of Texas Southwestern Medical School at Dallas and Parkland Hospital where he graduated in the top 2% of his class and was inducted into Alpha Omega Alpha, the medical honor society. He received his pediatric training at Children's Medical Center in Dallas. He is board certified in pediatrics and a fellow of the American Academy of Pediatrics (F.A.A.P.).

Dr. Young lives with his wife, Dana, and their three daughters Caitlyn, Christian, and Callan. They regularly attend Trinity Baptist Church and find meaning in life through their personal relationship with Jesus Christ.

"For God so loved the world that he gave his only Son, that whoever believes in him should not perish but have eternal life."
John 3:16

Contents

Warning — Disclaimer

Do NOT use the practices described in this book without first contacting your family physician or gynecologist. The practices in this book should only be performed under the direct guidance of a licensed medical doctor.

The practices described in this book cannot guarantee that you will conceive a child of the desired sex.

How To Have A Girl
Chapter I

I. Introduction

This book is designed to be a step-by-step quide that teaches specific practices which can maximize your chances of conceiving a female child. We cannot guarantee that you will have a baby girl, but, if the practices outlined in this book are accurately followed, research studies have proven that the probability of conceiving a female child will be increased.

A. Reasons for Desiring Sex Selection.

The reasons why people desire to conceive a child of a particular sex are infinite, and the factors which influence each person are unique. Since you are taking the time to read this book, we infer that you are interested in conceiving a daughter. Although you may feel very strongly about your preference, all of the factors which contribute to this desire may not be readily apparent to you. We feel that a full understanding of your motivational factors is healthy and will strengthen your resolve. Influencing the sex of your child is not a simple task, and, therefore, you must be committed to your goal. We will briefly discuss a few of the more common reasons for desiring preselection.

1. Two Children: 1 boy and 1 girl

The size of American families has been steadily declining during the past few decades. Early in this century, children were an economic necessity: after a short period of nurturing, they could be put to work to raise or maintain the family standard of living. Thus, large families were the rule rather than the exception. With such large numbers of children and almost equal numbers of males and females conceived, the chance of one sex not being represented was very remote. Times have changed. Children are now more of an economic liability. It is not uncommon for children to require economic assistance into their early 20's or beyond. Thus, couples often discuss children in terms of the number they are able to afford. Consequently, they want smaller families of 2 or 3 children, and the sex of the children becomes an important topic.

Most of our friends and acquaintances have expressed the desire for 2 children: one boy and one girl, although not necessarily in that order. When questioned about their reasons, they commonly describe this as a 'complete family'. They stress that boys and girls are socialized differently in our country, and they want to share in both of these different experiences. In addition, many prospective parents expressed particular interest in having a child of the same sex as themselves.

2. Family Pressure

Although most of us consider ourselves to be independent from our families, their pressure, both direct and indirect, can influence our decisions in life. In particular, family pressure can influence one's desire to have a child of a particular sex. We have found this situation to be most prominent in families in which there is only one son. There is often a tremendous burden placed on the 'only son' to continue having children until a grandson is conceived to carry on the family name. Family pressure may also be felt if one sex has predominated in the family. For example, families in which male children or grandchildren have predominated may exert significant pressure to have a female child.

3. Medical Reasons

The medical reasons for desiring a particular sex are less frequent but very compelling. The most common reason may be the presence of a defective gene on the X chromosome in a family. The resulting disorders are known as X-linked recessive disorders, and although female offspring can carry the defective gene, only male offspring will commonly display the disease. Such diseases include Duchenne muscular dystrophy and hemophilia. Hundreds of other diseases with this pattern of inheritance have been identified but they are very rare. Families which harbor these genes often desire female offspring who will less frequently exhibit the disease.

4. Additional Reasons

Two other reasons were commonly expressed to us. First, many couples expressed a desire to have a particular sex as the first born. Yet, both boys and girls were felt to be the ideal first child by different families. Some couples felt that the oldest child should be a male in order to offer some protection to the younger child or children. Others desired a girl as the oldest child because they felt that she could help raise younger children. Obviously, these views are integrated with stereotypic sex roles, but they were widespread among our friends and acquaintances. Second, one sex was desired because that sex was felt to be easier to raise. Again, there was considerable disagreement on which sex is easier to raise.

The chances are great that your reasons for desiring a child of a particular sex are not listed above. We encourage private discussions with your partner about your own reasons. In our experience, it has been helpful for each partner to write his or her individual reasons on a piece of paper and then discuss them together. Some couples may find that preselection is not important for the first pregnancy but becomes a larger issue in subsequent pregnancies. Others may find that the desire for a given sex is so overwhelming that each pregnancy should be influenced until a child of that sex is conceived. If both partners agree that a female child is desired, we hope that you will adeptly follow the methods in this book to increase your chance of conceiving a girl.

B. Priorities

Before we proceed into discussions about preselecting the sex of your next child, we feel compelled to state our position on the highest priority when planning a pregnancy:

THE HIGHEST PRIORITY IS THE DELIVERY OF A HEALTHY BABY

Our close association with pediatric patients over the past years has convinced us that a normal, healthy infant is the primary goal. Thus, if there is any chance that a preselection activity may hinder the health or development of the offspring, it should not be performed. We believe that the practices recommended in this book will have no adverse effect on the health or development of a new child; however, we encourage detailed discussions with your physician about participation in the methods presented in this book. If either partner or a trusted physician has any reservations about the methods presented here, the couple should employ medical procedures which can preselect sex or concentrate on conceiving a healthy child without regard to its sex.

C. Impact of Sex Preselection

Normal couples engaging in random intercourse will have an approximately equal chance of conceiving either a girl or a boy.

In other words, they have one chance in two of conceiving a child of either sex. We would like to possess a method of preselecting the gender of children which is easily performed at home and always yields the desired sex. Unfortunately, no such method exists. The majority of methods which can be used at home have not been supported by medical research, and most techniques which have been confirmed by research studies and significantly increase the conception of one sex require expensive procedures within medical laboratories. In contrast, when performed optimally, the method in this book, which can be performed at home without great expense, should be able to increase the probability of conceiving a female to well above that of the general population. Again, we cannot guarantee that you will have a child of the desired sex, but we can certainly increase your chances.

E. Organization of this Book

This book has been written for people with no background in medicine or science. Many of the terms we use will initially seem foreign, but we will attempt to define each new term as it arises. In addition, a glossary has been provided at the back of the book. We have arranged the information in outline form, and we hope that, as you begin to practice female sex preselection, you will be able to quickly find and reread any section of the material with which you are not entirely comfortable.

We will begin with a short discussion of the female menstrual cycle, and this will be followed by a discussion of the medical research over the past 25 years concerning sex preselection. The next seven chapters will discuss the methods which can be used at home to identify the time of ovulation. All of these methods will then be reviewed as we discuss female sex preselection. Finally, the last two chapters are devoted to further explanation of the calculations required and the sex preselection charts which will make preselection less complicated.

E. Caveats

1. Method Failures

As we have mentioned many times, no one can guarantee that you will conceive a child of a particular sex. If you are not prepared to love and care for a child of either sex, preselection methods should not be employed. We would instead recommend adoption in which the sex of the child can be more closely controlled.

2. Infertile Couples

This book is not designed for use by couples who have fertility problems. Although female sex preselection concentrates intercourse in the most fertile period of the menstrual cycle, there are many reasons for infertility other than the time or method of insemination. Thus, we recommend that couples with fertility problems contact their gynecologist and concentrate on the conception of a healthy child without regard to its sex.

"It is for us to make the effort. The result is always in God's hands."
Mohandas K. Gandhi

Chapter II

Basic Concepts

1. Determination of Males and Females

The sex of each new child is determined immediately at the time the sperm and egg unite. Both the sperm and the egg contain pieces of information known as sex chromosomes. Each egg contains one piece in the shape of an X which is called the X chromosome, but a sperm cell may have one in the shape of an X, like the egg, or a special piece in the shape of a Y, known as the Y chromosome. If the egg donates its X and the sperm also donates an X, the new child will have two X chromosomes and become a female.

Normal Female = XX

However, if the sperm which unites with the egg has a Y chromosome, the new child will have one X and one Y chromosome and become a male.

Normal Male = XY

It is the sex chromosome within the sperm that determines the sex of the child, and a Y chromosome will cause the child to be a boy. Since you desire to conceive a daughter, our goal will be to encourage the union of the egg with sperm which have an X chromosome.

2. Female Reproductive Tract

It is important that you become familiar with the organs of the female reproductive tract beginning with the ovaries and progressing to the external genitalia (see Fig. 2-1).

a. Ovaries

The ovaries are two, small organs located in the lower abdomen near the uterus — they are each roughly the size of a large almond. They are the female counterpart to the male testes and contain immature sex cells which can mature to form eggs. Normally, only one egg is released, or ovulated, from an ovary during each cycle. The cells which surround each developing egg are responsible for producing the two major female hormones: estrogen and progesterone. The egg and its surrounding cells are known as a follicle. Each follicle enlarges and moves to the surface of the ovary, and the release of the egg, known as ovulation, ruptures the capsule which surrounds the ovary. A pain in the lower abdomen is noted in up to 25% of women at the time of ovulation (Cunningham, 1993) — this pain has been named Mittleschmerz (see Chapter VIII).

b. Fallopian Tubes

The connections between the ovaries and the uterus are known as the oviducts or fallopian tubes. One tube lies on each side of the uterus. Each tube is composed of a muscular outer layer and a very delicate inner membrane which secretes mucus and has millions of hair-like projections known as cilia. The end of the tube next to the ovary has finger-like projections known as fimbria which act together to guide the egg into the tube after it has been expelled from the follicle of the ovary. Once captured by the fimbria, the egg begins to travel down the tube propelled by muscular contractions of the tube and rhythmic beating of the cilia toward the uterus. Although both mechanisms propel the egg down the tube, it does not travel directly toward the uterus but begins a gentle back and forth motion with a slow net movement toward the uterus — it usually takes a few days for an egg to migrate to the uterus after ovulation. Since an egg is thought to be viable for only 24 to 48 hours after ovulation, fertilization (the union of an egg and a sperm) normally occurs inside of the fallopian tubes. Notice that sperm must fight against the muscular contractions, the beating of the cilia, and the flow of mucus to reach the egg.

c. Uterus

The uterus, or womb, is the organ of the female reproductive tract which is responsible for receiving the fertilized egg, providing it with a place to implant, and providing nutrition and protection to the new child as it grows. It is approximately the size and shape of a pear and enlarges during puberty and after childbirth. The nonpregnant uterus has a small triangular cavity which can hold less than a teaspoon of fluid, but it is able to enlarge greatly to accommodate a full term infant. The walls consist of a thick outer layer of muscle and a thin inner membrane. The muscles of the wall are able to expand and are very strong; they will produce the contractions at the end of pregnancy which force the baby out through the birth canal. The inner lining is a specialized tissue capable of supporting a developing child. During each menstrual cycle, this membrane responds to estrogen and progesterone by becoming more thick with a rich blood supply in preparation for the implantation of a fertilized egg. If no pregnancy occurs, the inner portion of this membrane dies and is seen as a bloody discharge out of the vagina — menstrual flow or menstruation.

d. Cervix

The lower one-third of the uterus is known as the cervix. It is a thick, muscular tube with a thin inner canal which connects the uterus to the vagina. The opening to the canal from the vagina is known as the os; it is responsive to estrogen and becomes larger at the time of ovulation (see Chapter VII). The canal is lined with tiny glands which secrete mucus in response to estrogen; these secretions are initially thick and opaque, but, as the level of estrogen rises, they become profuse, clear, and elastic — this type of mucus has been called Spinnbarkeit and indicates that the time of ovulation is near (See Chapter VI).

e. Vagina

The vagina is a pliable tube designed to receive the human penis. It connects the cervix to the external genitalia, and it has a remarkable ability to distend which is exhibited at the time of childbirth. The vagina is populated by numerous bacteria which produce acid resulting in a hostile environment for yeast and other bacteria; these organisms would otherwise grow, populate the vagina, and cause discomfort. Unfortunately, this acid environment is also harmful for sperm.

3. The Menstrual Cycle

To influence the sex of your next child, it will be very important to know and recognize the changes which occur during the female menstrual cycle. Each menstrual cycle begins with the first day of menstrual flow and ends with the beginning of the next menstrual flow. The cycle can be broken down into three periods including the follicular phase, the time of ovulation, and the luteal phase (see Fig. 2-2). However, we will also discuss an additional segment of each menstrual cycle known as the fertile period — that period of time during which intercourse can with reasonable probability result in the fertilization of an egg.

Although the ideal menstrual cycle is considered to be 28 days, there is significant variation among women and between individual cycles in a given woman. Actually, only 15% of women have a 28 day cycle (Cunningham, 1993), but, for the purpose of learning the phases of the menstrual cycle, we will discuss only the ideal 28 day cycle.

a. Follicular phase

The first period of the menstrual cycle is known as the follicular phase and is composed of both menstruation and the proliferative phase.

$$\frac{\text{Menstruation} + \text{Proliferative Phase}}{= \text{Follicular Phase}}$$

It begins with the first day of menstruation and ends just prior to ovulation (see Fig. 2-2). This period of time has been named the follicular phase because, during this time, the follicle enlarges and matures in preparation for ovulation of a mature egg.

This phase is frequently 12 to 16 days but may vary from 8 to 20 days in normal women (Cunningham, 1993). In contrast, the luteal phase is usually very constant, and, thus, alterations in the length of a given menstrual cycle are usually due to variations in the length of its follicular phase. During this phase, Follicle Stimulating Hormone or FSH is secreted by the pituitary region of the brain; it causes the cells of the follicle to produce estrogen.

i. Menstruation

The first few days of the follicular phase are known as menstruation.

> **Menstruation is the periodic sloughing of the inner lining of the uterus as a bloody discharge; it occurs regularly from puberty until menopause.**

During each menstrual cycle, the uterine lining becomes prepared to accept and nurture a fertilized egg, but, when no fertilization occurs, this old lining is removed so that a fresh lining can be grown for the next ovulated egg. Menstrual flow usually lasts from 4 to 6 days, but lengths from 2 to 8 days may be seen in many women; while there is a significant variation in the length of flow, it is usually fairly constant from cycle to cycle in a given woman (Cunningham, 1993).

ii. Proliferative phase

The second part of the follicular phase is known as the proliferative phase; it begins with the end of menstruation and continues until just prior to ovulation. During this phase, the uterine inner lining begins to once again enlarge in preparation for ovulation. In addition, FSH acts on follicles to mature them in preparation for ovulation. Many follicles are initially stimulated, but, for reasons unknown at present, one follicle continues to enlarge while the remainder regress. The follicle enlarges by multiplication of the follicular cells around the egg, and, as the follicle enlarges, it moves closer to the surface of the ovary in preparation for ovulation. The follicular cells are also stimulated by FSH to secrete estrogens which have numerous effects on the female body including:

(1) growth of the inner lining of the uterus in preparation to accept a fertilized egg

(2) an increase in the production of clear and elastic cervical mucus

(3) an increase in the size of the opening (os) of the cervix

In addition, elevated levels of estrogen cause the pituitary gland of the brain to begin production of Luteinizing Hormone or LH which will induce ovulation.

b. Ovulation

The release of a mature egg from the ovaries is known as ovulation — this is the second major phase of the menstrual cycle (see Fig. 2-2). At the end of the proliferative phase, Luteinizing Hormone (LH) is secreted by the pituitary in response to increased levels of estrogen, and it causes ovulation: the wall of the follicle ruptures and the mature egg and its surrounding cells are gently released into the abdominal cavity.

The level of LH rises in the bloodstream and urine just prior to ovulation (see Chapter X).

The process of ovulation takes only 2 to 3 minutes. After ovulation, the egg is picked up by the finger-like projections (fimbria) of the fallopian tubes and begins its slow journey to the uterus.

c. Luteal Phase

The final phase of the menstrual cycle is known as the luteal phase; it begins just after ovulation and continues until just before the next menstruation begins (see Fig. 2-2). The LH surge which induced ovulation also causes the follicular cells to change from the production of estrogens to the production of progesterone. Therefore, a rise in progesterone is seen after the LH surge. Progesterone has two major functions:

> (1) it prepares the inner lining of the uterus to receive a fertilized egg

> and

> (2) if fertilization occurs, it must be secreted by the follicle cells which remain in the ovary during the first few weeks after implantation; the loss of this hormone would result in a spontaneous abortion.

In addition to these major effects, progesterone also causes an increase in the (basal) body temperature of the female and causes the production of cervical mucus to decrease — these changes have been used for many years to identify the time of ovulation (see Chapters V and VI).

The length of each luteal phase is very constant. The average length is 14 days—just as in the ideal cycle (Cunningham, 1993). However, we consider any length from 12 to 16 days to be within normal limits. Regardless of the absolute length of the luteal phase, it is usually the same length from cycle to cycle in a given woman. At the end of this phase, the level of progesterone begins to decrease. Without the support of progesterone, the inner lining of the uterus begins to die, and the next menstruation begins marking the end of the cycle.

d. Fertile Period

For those couples interested in conceiving a female child, the fertile period is the most important period of time during the menstrual cycle. It can be defined as follows:

> **The period of time during the menstrual cycle during which intercourse can with reasonable probability result in the fertilization of an egg.**

The most fertile time of the menstrual cycle occurs near the time of ovulation. If sexual intercourse could occur just minutes before the time of ovulation, sperm could travel up the female tract and congregate in the fallopian tubes awaiting the arrival of the newly ovulated egg; this would yield the highest probability of fertilization of the egg. However, intercourse both before and after this time can readily result in fertilization of the egg.

i. The fertile period - before ovulation

When insemination occurs prior to the time of ovulation, sperm migrate up the female tract and await the arrival of the egg. As time passes, some of the sperm will travel out of the fallopian tube into the abdominal cavity, some of the sperm will run out of energy and cease to swim, and others will lose their ability to fertilize an egg. For a short period of time after insemination, sperm will continue to migrate up the tract from the vagina, cervix, and uterus to replenish the wandering and dying sperm. In order to know how long before ovulation insemination can occur with a reasonable probability of fertilization, we must know the answer to the question:

*How long can sperm survive and remain fertile in
the female reproductive tract?*

Unfortunately, researchers do not agree about the absolute
length of sperm survival. Most would propose that sperm can
survive for many days in the female reproductive tract but only
retain the ability to fertilize an egg for 48 to 72 hours. However,
we do not agree with this concept. Studies have been performed
which examine the chance of conceiving a child on each day of
the menstrual cycle, and they have indicated that the probability
of conception may be elevated for up to 6 days prior to ovulation
(Royston, 1982). For the purpose of sex preselection, we will
consider the pre-ovulatory fertile period to be 6 days in length.
Thus, in the ideal menstrual cycle, the fertile period begins on day
8 (14-6=8) -- see Figure 2-2.

ii. The fertile period - after ovulation

There is less disagreement concerning the length of time after
ovulation during which intercourse can lead to fertilization.
After ovulation, the egg normally moves into the fallopian tube
where it waits for the arrival of a sperm. In order to determine
the length of this post-ovulatory fertile period, we must have an
answer to the question:

*How long after ovulation will the egg retain the
ability to successfully unite with sperm?*

Most researchers agree that the egg will degenerate after only 24
to 48 hours. For the purpose of sex preselection, we will consider
the post-ovulatory period to last 2 days. Thus, in the ideal
menstrual cycle, the fertile period will continue through day 16

(14+2) of the cycle. There may be an increased incidence of spontaneous abortion or malformations in pregnancies resulting from insemination after ovulation. Researchers have theorized that the more complex egg degenerates more quickly than sperm and this may lead to errors as the cells split into new cells. Although the evidence is not conclusive that there is an increase in either abortions or malformations, we recommend no intercourse during the post-ovulation fertile period.

4. Summary of Important Concepts

An understanding of the following general concepts will enhance your practice of sex preselection:

- Estrogen causes an increase in clear mucus production by the glands of the cervix and causes the opening of the cervix to enlarge.

- Pituitary LH induces ovulation and production of progesterone by the ovaries.

- LH rises in the bloodstream and urine just prior to ovulation.

- Progesterone causes the cervical glands to produce a small amount of thick mucus and the opening of the cervix to become smaller.

- Progesterone increases near the time of ovulation and causes an increase in the basal body temperature of the woman.

- The follicular phase may vary significantly in length.

- The luteal phase is usually more constant in length and lasts 12 to 16 days in most women.

- Variations in cycle length are usually due to alterations in the length of the follicular phase — the time before ovulation.

- We consider the fertile period to begin 6 days prior to ovulation and end 2 days after ovulation.

- Do **NOT** have intercourse during the first two or three days after ovulation.

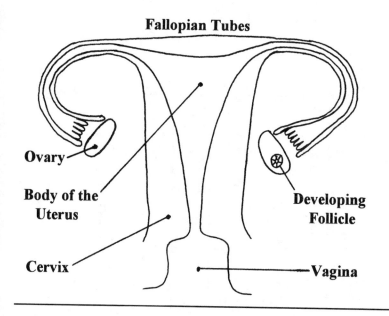

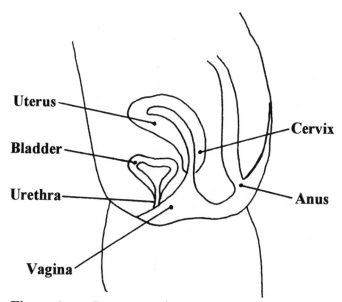

Figure 2-1: Organs of the Female Reproductive Tract

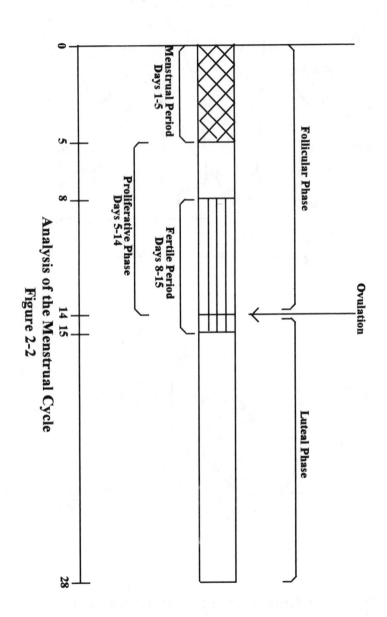

Analysis of the Menstrual Cycle
Figure 2-2

Chapter III

Current Research

"We shall seek the truth and endure the consequences."
Charles Seymour

Before the advent of scientific research, couples followed myths and old wives tales which claimed to influence the sex of offspring. These practices were usually initiated because they appeared logical, were performed by a couple who had many children of one sex, or were consistent with beliefs held strongly by the participants. Couples who received the sex of child that they desired often became very vocal supporters of the practice. In contrast, couples who delivered the opposite sex often thought or were told that they did not perform the activity appropriately, and, even if they felt that the practice had no effect on the sex of their child, they rarely denounced it with the fervor of the couples who had received their desired girl or boy. Thus, couples often performed bizarre rituals at the time of intercourse in order to influence the sex of their next child.

Today, scientists attempt to study as many conceptions as possible to remove the element of chance and find those practices which truly alter the ratio of males to females at birth. We will briefly discuss, in chronological order, the significant research concerning sex preselection which has been performed during the past three decades.

1. Shettles' Proposals

The first widely read author to present a scientific method of altering the sex ratio at birth was Dr. Landrum B. Shettles. Along with David Rorvik, he published a book in 1970 titled "Your Baby's Sex: Now You Can Choose." The following tenets of his book became very widely known through extensive media coverage:

> *To increase the probability of female offspring, insemination should occur 2 or more days before ovulation, with acidic douches, using the missionary position, and without female orgasm.*

> *To increase the probability of male offspring, insemination should occur as close to the time of ovulation as possible, with non-acidic douches, using the rear entry position, and with female orgasm.*

Although he first published these proposals over twenty years ago, we have found that they are firmly entrenched in the general knowledge of the population: when we first expressed an interest in sex preselection, the advice of our relatives and friends closely approximated Shettles' proposals. In addition, couples we have met in the past two years have confided that they possess a copy of his book and plan to follow it to conceive their next child.

We can summarize the concepts behind Dr. Shettles proposals as follows:

He felt that X-bearing (female) sperm were able to remain viable longer and withstand more stress than the Y-bearing (male) sperm. Thus, he reasoned:

- insemination many days before ovulation would favor the more hardy female sperm who would survive longer.

- prolonged contact with the acid environment of the vagina would favor the hardy X-bearing sperm; thus, acid douches were thought to predispose to female offspring.

- the missionary position was recommended because it was felt to increase the degree of sperm contact with the vaginal secretions.

He felt that Y-bearing sperm were weaker and less able to withstand stress. However, because of their shape and lower weight, he concluded that they were faster.

-if all conditions were equal and an egg were waiting to be fertilized, he felt that the faster Y-bearing sperm would reach it first; thus, he recommended insemination at ovulation.

- he recommended non-acidic (basic) douches to protect the weaker Y-bearing sperm from the normally acidic vaginal environment.

- he recommended the rear entry position because he felt it would decrease the degree of contact with the vaginal secretions.

- female orgasms were also thought to result in a less acidic vaginal environment.

Shettles' beliefs were supported by his personal experience with artificial insemination in which insemination at the time of ovulation yielded a high percentage of males. Researchers, for some time after the publication of his book, continued to find that artificial insemination at the time of ovulation yielded a higher percentage of males. Unfortunately for Dr. Shettles and the millions who followed his proposals, however, the results from artificial insemination do not correlate with those from natural insemination. In fact, they are in direct opposition. Numerous studies, which will be discussed in the next section, have demonstrated a preponderance of female births with natural insemination at the time of ovulation and more male births with natural insemination days prior to or after ovulation. Unknowingly, his recommendations for the timing of intercourse lowered the probability of success.

"The best laid plans of mice and men oft' gang agley."
Robert Burns

2. Current Research

The only method of home sex preselection firmly supported by current research is alteration of the time of insemination relative to ovulation. In the first column of Figure 3-1, we have listed the major research studies over the past 25 years which have investigated the sex of children born at different times relative to ovulation. The middle columns of Figure 3-1 list the findings of each study divided into the percentage of male and female births with insemination "near" or "far" from ovulation. The studies usually concur on the definition of intercourse "near" ovulation but, unfortunately, these studies have each defined the concept of "far" differently. For example, some of the studies did not consider any insemination over 2 days before ovulation to be capable of resulting in the fertilization of an egg — their "far" group included only births from insemination 2 days before and 2 days after ovulation. In contrast, other studies considered insemination up to 6 days prior to ovulation as part of the "far" group. Thus, we cannot merely discuss the results in this table, but, instead, we must look carefully at each study to find out what they reveal about sex preselection.

Finally, the third column lists the results of any statistical analysis which was performed on the research data. This analysis determines the probability that the study results could have occurred by chance. Studies are designated as "statistically significant" if the statistical analysis determines that there is less than a 5% chance that the study results occurred by random chance or luck.

> **Statistically significant = less than a 5% chance that the study results occurred by random chance.**

The significance of a study is closely tied to the number of participants in the study — as more couples are studied, the chance that the study results occurred by chance tends to decrease.

In general, the studies in Figure 3-1 support the concept that insemination on those days near ovulation will result in more female offspring, while insemination either many days before or after ovulation will result in more male offspring:

More girls are conceived near ovulation.

More boys are conceived away from ovulation.

a. Guerrero

In 1974, Rodrigo Guerrero published landmark studies concerning the day of insemination in relation to ovulation. Unlike previous research in this area, he studied data from natural and artificial insemination separately. In addition, instead of studying only the day of the menstrual cycle in which insemination occurred, he studied insemination relative to the day of ovulation as determined by basal body temperature (BBT) charting. BBT charting is a widely used method of contraception that relies on changes in body temperature with the menstrual cycle to determine ovulation; the BBT shifts from low to high during a normal menstrual cycle and ovulation occurs near the temperature shift.

Dr. Guerrero studied the BBT charts of 875 couples in which pregnancy had occurred. He designated the day of ovulation by the BBT charts as Day 0 and numbered other days of the menstrual cycle accordingly. For example, the day prior to ovulation was designated as day -1. He then correlated the births which occurred due to insemination on a given day and calculated the percentage of male births. Please see Figure 3-2 which summarizes his findings. Notice that the percentage of female births is highest at the time of ovulation and decreases steadily as insemination becomes more distant from ovulation. The lower percentage of female births which occurred in the days prior to ovulation and after ovulation proved to be statistically significant; once again, this means that the chance of these results occurring randomly was less than 5% — in fact, since he was able to study the BBT charts of such a large number of couples, statistical analysis found that there was less than a 0.1% chance that the results occurred by accident.

b. Harlap

Susan Harlap studied this subject and published her results in 1979 in the New England Journal of Medicine. She studied 3,658 births to Jewish women who practiced niddah — the orthodox ritual of sexual separation. Couples who practice niddah abstain from sex during the first 7 days after the cessation of menses. Later in the seventh day, each woman visits a bath house, has a ritual bath, and then returns home to have intercourse. With such a prolonged period of abstinence, most couples have an increase in sexual activity during the first few days after niddah. Menstrual flow lasts 4 to 6 days in the majority of women which would place the first day of intercourse from day 11 (4 + 7) to day 13 (6 + 7). In the ideal 28 day cycle with ovulation on day 14 and in many non-ideal cycles, intercourse would be concentrated at a very fertile period of the menstrual cycle. Thus, niddah, in a population of women not practicing contraception, would help to increase the probability of fertilization.

Her results revealed the same general pattern reported by Guerrero: more females conceived at the time of ovulation and more males conceived 2 or more days before and after ovulation. Her findings on the days prior to ovulation were not as striking with only 47% female babies born when intercourse occurred 2 days before the expected day of ovulation. However, she found an impressive 34% female births when conception occurred 2 days after ovulation. She found the same pattern in women regardless of age, height, weight, social class, educational level, or ethnic group.

Her results were very consistent with those of Guerrero. The period beginning 2 days after ovulation was associated with a very low percentage of female births. Unfortunately, she discarded information from women who had intercourse more than 2 days prior to ovulation from consideration — she felt that these women had not remembered the events around fertilization correctly. In Guerrero's study, the probability of female offspring only decreased to below 50% when insemination occurred more than 2 days before ovulation (see Fig. 3-2). Thus, her finding of approximately 50% females born with insemination 2 days prior to ovulation is precisely what we would expect, and her study does not confirm nor refute Guerrero's observations of fewer females being conceived 3 or more days before ovulation.

c. France et al

In 1984, John France and associates published a study of this topic in Fertility and Sterility, a medical journal. They set out to test the theory of Shettles, but, instead of merely looking back at the records of couples who had achieved pregnancy, they enrolled 185 couples who desired to preselect sex in their study and followed them until they conceived or dropped out of the study. Each couple was instructed in basal body temperature recording and identification of fertile cervical mucus, and urine was collected daily near ovulation to test for luteinizing hormone (LH). In order to test Shettles theory, couples who desired a boy were instructed to have intercourse at the time of ovulation while couples who desired a girl were instructed to have intercourse 2 to 3 days prior to ovulation. They were asked to begin abstinence from day 7 of the cycle or when mucus symptoms were first noted, have only one act of intercourse in the fertile period, and then abstain until at least 5 days after the most fertile mucus discharge was noted. A total of 57 pregnancies were identified of which 52 went to term with the delivery of a child. Unfortunately, 19 babies had to be removed from the study because their parents had more than one act of intercourse in the fertile period. Thus, 33 infants were conceived with a single, verifiable insemination during the fertile period. France then compared the day of insemination with the time of ovulation as determined by BBT charting, appearance of the peak mucus symptom, and urinary LH testing.

Relating insemination to the peak of cervical mucus production produced significant results. Males were produced by insemination from day -6 to day 0, and females resulted when insemination occurred only from day -3 to day +1. Using this indicator of ovulation, only 25% of the males were conceived by sperm which had been in the female tract two or fewer days. Also, notice that insemination 4 or more days prior to ovulation yielded no female offspring.

Only 39% of the couples conceived a child of the sex that they desired while following Shettles' proposals. Remember that with only random intercourse we would expect approximately 50% of the couples to receive a child of the desired sex. Thus, following Shettles' theory actually decreased their probability of success. This clearly contradicts the proposals of Shettles and offers strong support for the findings of Guerrero and Harlap.

d. World Health Organization

The World Health Organization or WHO is a group which scientifically studies ways in which the health and quality of life of people throughout the world can be improved. They are very concerned with overpopulation and have promoted the use of natural family planning (NFP) techniques to decrease fertility in developing countries. These techniques concentrate on identifying the most fertile period of the menstrual cycle and avoiding intercourse at that time. They have sponsored numerous research studies concerning NFP, and, in 1984, they published a study which dealt with the outcome of pregnancy after the use of NFP techniques.

They performed a study which included patients from New Zealand, India, Ireland, Philippines, and El Salvador. A total of 163 pregnancies occurred during the study in which the outcome of the pregnancy was known. Although the babies born to the participants included only 42% females, which is lower than the 49% females seen in the general population, they did find more females, 45%, born within 1 day of the Peak Day and fewer born both before and after ovulation: 39% conceived 2 to 5 days before ovulation and 33% conceived 2 to 4 days after ovulation. Although these results are consistent with Guerrero's observations, they were unable to pass the statistical tests required to be considered significant.

e. Simcock

In 1985, Barbara W. Simcock published a study, similar to the France study, in the Medical Journal of Australia. She, likewise, set out to study the effect of a modified Shettles theory. She enrolled women who wanted to preselect the sex of their next child and taught them how to follow basal body temperatures (BBTs). For three consecutive cycles, each woman used non-hormonal birth control and took daily temperatures. At the end of this time, she reviewed the temperature charts and designated the day prior to the temperature shift in past cycles as the estimated day of ovulation in the next cycle. In conjunction with Shettles' theory, those women who desired a son were instructed to have intercourse on the estimated day of ovulation (Day 0) and used a mildly alkaline douche; conversely, those women who desired a daughter were instructed to have intercourse 3 days prior to ovulation (Day -3) and used a mildly acidic douche. Although she conducted her study for four years (1979 - 1983), only 73 pregnancies with 67 live births occurred by women who correctly followed her instructions.

Her results could have occurred by chance — they were not statistically significant — but they are interesting to examine. Insemination near ovulation yielded 19 live infants with 63% females and 37% males. Simcock found an even more pronounced predisposition for females at the time of ovulation than Guerrero found in his studies. It is somewhat more interesting to compare her findings with insemination away from ovulation with the findings of Guerrero. She chose to have couples who desired girls inseminate 3 days prior to ovulation (Day -3). These couples delivered 48 live infants of which 52% were male and 48% were female. She concluded that the success rate for preselection away from ovulation was only 50% — no change from random insemination. However, once again, compare her results to Guerrero's 1974 study in Figure 3-2; her finding of 48% female births would lie almost exactly on this curve and support his findings. In order to attempt to influence the sex of the offspring, she should have instructed her couples to have sex at least 4 and possibly more days prior to ovulation. We can see that the findings of Dr. Simcock are in direct opposition to Dr. Shettles' theory and support the observations of Dr. Guerrero.

f. Perez et al

Dr. Perez and associates of Santiago, Chile were also intrigued by the study of Dr. France and performed a study of this topic in 1985. They reviewed 114 conception charts from women who used natural family planning techniques. In 52 charts, the act of conception which resulted in fertilization could be identified between Day -6 and Day +3. They designated two different time periods. First, they labelled Day 0 and Day -1 as the 'most fertile days'. Next, they labelled the time periods from Day -6 to Day -2 and from Day +1 to Day +3 as the 'less fertile days'. On the 'most fertile days', they found 63% females conceived, while on the 'less fertile days' 24% of children conceived were female. Their results were highly significant on statistical tests, and further confirmed Guerrero's findings.

The previous six studies clearly support a change in the sex ratio dependent upon the time of insemination. Zarutskie and associates in 1989 examined these studies and concluded, as we have, that the sex ratio changes in relation to insemination as described by Guerrero. Unfortunately, they did not feel that this change is of sufficient magnitude to be useful by average couples. We strongly disagree. These studies indicate that intercourse very near to the time of ovulation would increase the probability of conceiving a female to greater than 60% for each pregnancy. **We feel that, with meticulous determination of ovulation and carefully planned intercourse, the sex ratio at birth can be significantly altered by couples in their own home.**

3. Important Concepts and Recommendations

> **Insemination on Days 0 or -1 will produce the greatest chance of conceiving a girl.**
>
> **Intercourse should be planned during the 72 hour period from Day -1 to Day +1.**

4. Importance of the Exact Determination of Ovulation

Home sex preselection is based on the accurate determination of ovulation and the educated estimation of the time of ovulation in upcoming cycles. The time of ovulation must be accurately known in order for the female period to be identified. In the following chapters, we will discuss many methods for determining ovulation which can be used in your own home.

Chapter IV - Calendar Method
Chapter V - Basal Body Temperature Graphing
Chapter VI - Cervical Mucus Determinations
Chapter VII - Cervical Observation
Chapter VIII - Mittleschmerz
Chapter IX - Cervical Chemistry
Chapter X - Urinary LH Testing

"A lasting work requires extensive preparation."
Douglas Rumford

Figure 3-1
Natural Insemination Time vs. Ovulation

STUDY	TIME OF INSEMINATION			STATISTICS
	NEAR	FAR		
Guerrero 1974	43%M 57%F	68%M 32%F		Very Significant p < 0.1%
Harlap 1979	49%M 51%F	-2 days: 53%M 47%F	+2 days: 66%M 34%F	Significant p < 2.5%
France 1984	36%M 64%F	68%M 32%F		Cervical Mucus Study Significant p < 5.0%
WHO 1984	51%M 49%F	>-2 days: 61%M 39%F	>+2 days: 67%M 33%F	Not Significant
Simcock 1985	37%M 63%F	52%M 48%F		Not Significant p < 7.5%
Perez 1985	37%M 63%F	76%M 24%F		Highly Significant

Figure 3-2

Risk of Female Conception by Cycle Day

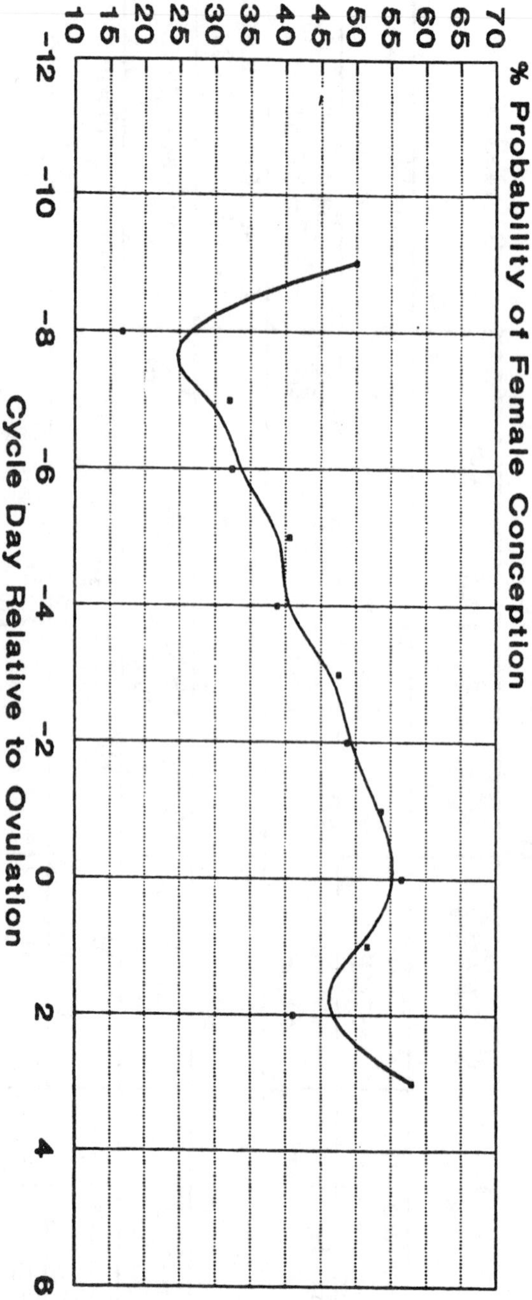

% Probability of Female Conception

Cycle Day Relative to Ovulation

Adapted from R. Guerrero, NEJM, 1974

Chapter IV

Calendar Method

1. Introduction

The Calendar Method for determining the fertile period and time of ovulation has been in use since the early 1930's. The Rhythm Method of birth control, which was advocated by the Catholic Church for many years, is based on calendar recording. The key to this method of determining ovulation is that:

The luteal phase of the menstrual cycle is very constant.

In other words, the interval from ovulation to the next menstruation is very constant; it lasts 14 days in many women, but any length from 12 to 16 days will be found in a large number of women. The length of the luteal phase, whether 12, 14, or 16 days, is constant in most women across cycles. We all know that the length of the menstrual cycle can vary considerably, but, in most cases, it is the time before ovulation, known as the follicular phase, which is becoming longer or shorter. In fact, the follicular phase can become unexpectedly lengthened in a woman who is subjected to any type of physical or emotional stress.

In the original Calendar Method, the Luteal Phase Length (**LPL**) was estimated to be 14 days in all women who practiced it. Each woman would mark her first day of each menstrual period on the calendar, and the Menstrual Cycle Length (**MCL**) for the upcoming cycle was estimated by looking at the length of the previous cycle or cycles on her calendar. The Day of

Ovulation (**DO**) in the next cycle was then calculated by subtracting 14 from the estimated Menstrual Cycle Length:

$$\text{MCL} = \textbf{Menstrual Cycle Length}$$
$$\text{LPL} = \textbf{Luteal Phase Length} = 14$$
$$\text{DO} = \textbf{Day of Ovulation}$$

$$\textbf{DO} = \textbf{MCL} - 14$$

In an ideal cycle:

$$\text{MCL} = 28 \text{ days}$$
$$\text{LPL} = 14 \text{ days}$$

$$\text{DO} = 28 - 14$$
$$= 14$$

Therefore, ovulation would be expected on day 14 of an ideal cycle.

This DO was marked clearly on the calendar. The couples would then abstain from intercourse for a specific number of days both before and after ovulation in order to prevent pregnancy, and these days were also clearly marked. The length of abstinence varied according to both the person who instructed the couple and the individuals themselves, but it was common for couples to consider 6 days before and 2 or 3 days after the Day of Ovulation to be fertile days.

Example 4-1 — Traditional Calendar Method

> Bill and Hillary are a couple who are having intercourse and have decided to use the traditional Calendar Method as a form of birth control. They obtain a calendar and begin to mark the first day of

each menstrual period on the proper day. After the second menstrual period is recorded on the calendar, they are able to calculate the previous cycle length. It lasted 28 days. Using an estimate of 14 days for the LPL, they then calculate the expected day of ovulation to be day 14. They next calculate the days of the fertile period: those days which begin 6 days before ovulation and end 3 days after ovulation.

$$\text{First day} = 14 - 6 = 8$$
$$\text{Last day} = 14 + 3 = 17$$

The first day of menstrual flow is designated as day 1 of each cycle. They may have unprotected intercourse from day 1 through 7 and day 18 through the end of the cycle, but they must abstain during the fertile period — days 8 through 17.

After observing several cycles, they find that Hillary's cycles are actually 30 days in length and very regular. They recalculate the Day of Ovulation (DO) based on this new MCL:

$$DO = 30 - 14$$
$$= 16$$

Then, they recalculate the fertile period:

$$\text{First day} = 16 - 6 = 10$$
$$\text{Last day} = 16 + 3 = 19$$

They consequently abstain on days 10 through 19 in each upcoming cycle to avoid conception within the fertile period. This period lasts only 10 days or approximately one-third of each cycle, and they have little difficulty complying with the method.

Obviously, the traditional Calendar Method is a poor way of estimating the Day of Ovulation because there are two possible sources of error. First, the next menstrual cycle may be much longer or shorter than the previous cycle. And, second, the luteal phase of the woman in question may not be exactly 14 days. For these two reasons and because of unplanned intercourse during the fertile period, this method had a high failure rate.

Women, such as Hillary, who have regular menstrual cycles should not have the first source of error discussed above. Barring unsuspected prolongation of the follicular phase, they should have a good estimate of the MCL in the next cycle. However, women with irregular cycles have searched for a way to improve the efficiency of this method. They increased its efficiency by increasing the number of days of abstinence. They would calculate an estimated Day of Ovulation based not on the previous or average MCL but on both the shortest and longest possible MCL. Using the DO from the shortest MCL they would subtract 6 days and consider this the first possible fertile day. Then, they would use the DO calculated from the longest MCL, move 3 days past this date, and consider this day the last possible fertile day. The couples would, ideally, abstain on all days between the first and last fertile days. These calculations did improve the identification of the fertile period, but it narrowed the possible days of intercourse to such an extent that many couples were unable to follow it.

Example 4-2 — Irregular Cycles

George and Barbara are planning to use the traditional Calendar Method for birth control. Unfortunately, Barbara has irregular cycles lasting

28 to 32 days. The majority of this variation should be due to changes in the follicular phase length. Ovulation occurs earliest in the 28 day or shortest cycle:

$$\text{Short Cycle DO} = 28 - 14$$
$$= 14$$

The beginning of the fertile period is then calculated from the earliest possible ovulation:

$$\text{First day} = 14 - 6 = 8$$

Ovulation occurs at the latest time in the longest cycle:

$$\text{Long Cycle DO} = 32 - 14$$
$$= 18$$

The last possible fertile day can then be calculated:

$$\text{Last day} = 18 + 3$$
$$= 21$$

Thus, George and Barbara must stop intercourse on day 7 and not resume until day 21 — a total of 15 days or approximately one-half of the cycle. This longer period of abstinence in irregular cycles greatly reduces compliance.

Both women with regular and irregular cycles were able to improve the Calendar Method by reducing error in the estimation of the Luteal Phase Length (LPL). As we mentioned earlier, the luteal phase is constant across cycles in most women. The original method chose 14 days because it is the average length, but it may be several days longer or shorter than the phase in the woman in question. In order to find the length of her own luteal phase, each woman would use another home method, such as basal body temperature changes or the presence of pain near ovulation, to identify ovulation. They would identify the presumed day of ovulation (DO) on their calendar and, at the end of the cycle, calculate the LPL using the following formula:

$$LPL = MCL - DO$$

Example 4-3 — Identification of the LPL

> Ron and Nancy are also practicing the traditional Calendar Method as a form of birth control. Nancy has regular menstrual cycles of 30 days. In order to calculate the Luteal Phase Length (LPL), they first must identify the Day of Ovulation (DO) using a second method. Nancy has a lower abdominal pain near the time of ovulation (Mittleschmerz) which indicated that ovulation occurred on cycle day 14. They then calculated Nancy's LPL in the previous cycle:

$$
\begin{aligned}
LPL &= MCL - DO \\
&= 30 - 14 \\
&= 16
\end{aligned}
$$

> Thus, Nancy's actual LPL is 2 days longer than the estimated LPL of the traditional Calendar Method. They will estimate that ovulation will occur on day 14 in the next cycle. The fertile period can then be calculated:

$$
\begin{aligned}
\text{First day} &= 14 - 6 = 8 \\
\text{Last day} &= 14 + 3 = 17
\end{aligned}
$$

In the women with regular menstrual periods, the Calendar Method was able to reasonably predict the day of ovulation. Conversely, irregular menstrual periods made prediction of the day of ovulation much less reliable and made contraception much more difficult because of marked restrictions on intercourse.

2. Calculation : Day of Ovulation

Unlike the women described above who were using the Calendar Method to avoid pregnancy, we want to use it to more precisely identify the time of ovulation and the beginning of the fertile period. The day of ovulation can be accurately estimated prior to the cycle if two conditions are met:

1. The menstrual cycles are regular.

2. The luteal phase length is calculated and is constant.

Unfortunately, few women will satisfy both of these conditions.

With an ideal cycle, ovulation occurs exactly half way through the cycle — this ideal state is discussed regularly and gives people the idea that ovulation always occurs at the middle of the cycle. Actually, very few women will ovulate exactly at mid-cycle.

Example 4-4 — Preselection and Regular Cycles

Bill and Hillary are now planning to practice sex preselection and desire a baby girl. Over the past months, they have closely followed Hillary's menstrual cycles. She has regular menstruation with cycles lasting 30 days. In addition, her luteal phases have consistently lasted 13 days — ovulation has been identified 13 days prior to the next menstrual period. Since Hillary has regular cycle lengths and luteal phase lengths, they can reliably estimate the expected day of ovulation in the upcoming cycle:

$$\begin{aligned} DO &= MCL - LPL \\ &= 30 - 13 \\ &= 17 \end{aligned}$$

In women with truly regular cycles, this method alone may be adequate for performing home sex preselection. Couples with irregular cycles should, however, also become proficient at this method because it can help them to become more observant at the proper time in the cycle.

Example 4-5 — Preselection and Irregular Cycles

George and Barbara are also planning to practice sex preselection and want to have a baby girl. In following Barbara's menstrual cycles, they have noted cycle lengths of 28 to 32 days. In contrast, her luteal phases have consistently lasted 14 days. We can calculate the possible ovulation days based on the range of menstrual cycle lengths:

$$\begin{aligned} \text{Short cycle } DO &= MCL - LPL \\ &= 28 - 14 \\ &= 14 \end{aligned}$$

$$\begin{aligned} \text{Long cycle } DO &= MCL - LPL \\ &= 32 - 14 \\ &= 18 \end{aligned}$$

Thus, with her irregular cycles, the Calendar Method can only predict that her ovulation will occur between days 14 to 18 of the next cycle. This is a wide variation, and, when used alone, this method would not be very helpful for influencing the baby's sex. Again, the Calendar Method can only reliably predict the day of ovulation when cycles are regular. This calculation will, however, be somewhat useful for George and Barbara because they will be more observant on Days 14 through 18 — it will be easier for them to recognize other signs and symptoms of ovulation.

3. Calculation : Fertile Period

We will now calculate the beginning of the period of fertility. As we discussed in Chapter II, we will consider the fertile period to begin 6 days prior to the day of ovulation:

FP = First Day of the Fertile Period

FP = DO - 6

This calculation is very important for you since you desire a female child. In Chapter III, we discussed research which indicated that the probability of conceiving a male is highest far from ovulation — at the very beginning of the fertile period; thus, intercourse must cease at the beginning of this period, and couples must begin to watch for evidence of ovulation.

Example 4-6 — Fertile Period with Regular Cycles

Since Bill and Hillary from Examples 4-1 and 4-4 want a baby girl, they would want to cease intercourse at the beginning of the fertile period — 4 to 6 days prior to the day of ovulation. We can calculate the first day of the fertile period:

$$FP = DO - 6$$
$$= 17 - 6$$
$$= 11$$

Therefore, they would cease intercourse on day 11 of the next menstrual cycle.

Again, since Hillary has perfectly regular cycles, the Calendar Method alone may allow them to influence the sex of their next child. Couples who have irregular cycles should, however, continue to follow the method because it will indicate the most probable days upon which the fertile period will begin. On these days, they can increase their level of awareness and perceive the slightest physical changes.

Example 4-7 — Fertile Period with Irregular Cycles

Since George and Barbara want a baby girl, they too would cease intercourse at the beginning of the fertile period. Calculation, however, with irregular cycles must use both the Short cycle DO and the Long cycle DO:

$$\text{Short cycle FP} = \text{Short cycle DO} - 6$$
$$= 14 - 6$$
$$= 8$$

$$\text{Long cycle FP} = \text{Long cycle DO} - 6$$
$$= 18 - 6$$
$$= 12$$

Our calculations indicate that the fertile period will begin at some time between days 8 and 12 of the next cycle. Since this spans 4 days of the next cycle and we consider the entire fertile period to be only 6 days prior to ovulation, the Calendar Method is, again, not extremely useful when the cycles are markedly irregular. Yet, George and Barbara can become more observant on Days 8 through 12 and more easily recognize the early signs and symptoms of the fertile period.

Our examples have used Hillary and Nancy, whom have perfectly regular cycles of equal length, and Barbara who has up to 4 days difference in the lengths of her menstrual cycles. The cycles do not have to be perfectly regular for the information to be valuable, but differences of 2 or more days decrease the value of this method significantly.

When discussing the fertile period, we must point out that fertilization can occur if intercourse takes place within 24 to 48 hours after ovulation. As noted in the previous chapter, fertilization at this time would result in a higher number of male births. In addition, we have not included this time period in our fertile period because this would violate our first priority: fertilization after ovulation may be associated with a higher incidence of spontaneous abortion. Thus, we discourage planned fertilization after ovulation. If the rhythm method is used for contraception during sex preselection, abstain for at least 2 or, preferably, 3 days after ovulation.

4. Improvement on the Traditional Calendar Method

Knowledge of the average phase and cycle lengths can improve the estimation of ovulation by the Calendar Method. In fact, in women with only occasionally irregular cycles, the estimations can be quite accurate. We have included a worksheet for calculation of the average values — the Cycle Summary Calculation Sheet or CSCS. It is located immediately in front of the monthly charts. The following information should be recorded at the top of each monthly chart and on the CSCS:

MCL = Menstrual Cycle Length
DO = Day of Ovulation
LPL = Luteal Phase Length
FP = First Day of Fertile Period

After this information for each cycle has been recorded, the average values can then be calculated:

ACL = Average Cycle Length
ADO = Average Day of Ovulation
ALPL = Average Luteal Phase Length
AFP = Average First day of Fertile Period

The formula for calculating each of these averages can be found in Chapter XIII. The first 3 columns of the CSCS are designed to record the observed values while the final 3 columns are reserved for the calculated values. Each averaged value is obtained by adding all of the observed values and dividing by the number of cycles over which the values were obtained:

$$\frac{\text{Sum of all values}}{\text{Number of cycles}}$$

By definition, average values are not calculated in the first cycle, but they should be calculated for each cycle thereafter. **The ADO is the best predictor of the day of ovulation in the next cycle.**

Example 4-8 — Improved Calendar Method

Jimmy and Rosalyn are a couple who are trying to conceive a girl. They have been following her menstrual cycles closely and graphing the values on her CSCS. It reveals that her shortest cycle was 27 days and her longest cycle was 36 days — a large degree of variability. We would initially assume that the Calendar Method would be of little value to them in influencing the sex of their child. However, placing the information on her CSCS allowed her to quickly see that one cycle was uncharacteristically short and that another cycle was inordinately long when compared to the 5 other cycles. They calculated her ADO to be 19.6 days. Thus, they planned intercourse between days 19 and 20 in the next cycle.

After the ADO has been identified, we can easily calculate the Average First Day of the Fertile Period (AFP):

$$AFP = ADO - 6$$

Example 4-9 — Calculation of the AFP

Since Jimmy and Rosalyn desire a daughter, they plan to cease intercourse at the beginning of the fertile period. They calculate the AFP as follows:

$$
\begin{aligned}
AFP &= ADO - 6 \\
&= 15.6 - 6 \\
&= 9.6
\end{aligned}
$$

In the next cycle, they plan to have intercourse immediately at the time of ovulation.

We have used these average values to refine the traditional Calendar Method. Calculation of the ALPL allows you to define the near constant LPL value for the particular woman practicing sex preselection. In addition, estimation of the upcoming cycle length by calculation of the ACL is more accurate than assuming a 28 day cycle. Women with perfectly regular cycles have no real need to calculate average values. However, women with some degree of irregularity in their cycles will be able to calculate the ADO and predict the next DO with more accuracy.

Although we have used each cycle length in calculation of the ACL, this is a matter of individual choice. In women with occasional long or short cycles, a couple could opt to discard both the longest and shortest cycles for calculation of the ACL. We would not recommend ignoring values until at least 6 cycles have been observed.

"When you can measure what you are speaking about, and express it in numbers, you know something about it; but when you cannot measure it, when you cannot express it in numbers, your knowledge is of a meager and unsatisfactory kind; it may be the beginning of knowledge, but you have scarcely, in your thoughts, advanced to the stage of science."
William Thomson, Lord Kelvin

Chapter V

Basal Body Temperature Graphing

1. Introduction

The basal body temperature or **BBT** is the temperature of the body at rest; it measures the heat generated by the body as it expends energy to keep the cells of the body alive. This includes the work of breathing and the work of the heart as it pumps blood rich in oxygen and nutrients to each cell of the body. By definition, it is the temperature of the body when it is inactive; activity entails the use of muscles which generate heat and increase the body temperature. The BBT is significantly influenced by hormones which circulate in the bloodstream, and, thus, changes in the hormone status of the body can be identified by the presence of changes in the BBT.

Graphs of daily basal body temperature have now been used for many years to avoid conception and to identify ovulation in couples with fertility problems. This method can be helpful for home sex preselection and is easily performed. It will play a significant role in sex preselection, and we will, therefore, discuss it in detail.

Figure 5-1: Classical BBT Graph

This graph depicts a basal body temperature curve constructed from daily BBT measurements.

> The temperature is initially lower, but, near midcycle, the temperature rises and is maintained at a higher level. This change in BBT near midcycle is known as the <u>BBT rise</u> or <u>BBT shift</u> and is felt to occur just shortly after ovulation.

To understand why the temperature rises after ovulation, we must return to our discussions of female hormone changes in Chapter II. Estrogen rises to high levels during the first half of the cycle. The pituitary region of the brain recognizes this and switches from the production of FSH to the production of LH or Luteinizing Hormone. LH causes the follicle to rupture (known as ovulation) and causes the follicular cells to produce progesterone; this hormone causes the body temperature to increase.

Progesterone causes the BBT to rise.

Progesterone rises after ovulation. Thus, the temperature rise will be detected shortly after ovulation.

Although the BBT rises in each ovulating woman, the change is small and, therefore, not readily recognized. In addition, the heat generated from movement after awakening further obscures or surpasses the BBT rise. Most women find that their oral temperature during the first half of the cycle is slightly higher than 97.0F. Moghissi in 1980 studied 10 women and found the average BBT prior to the rise near ovulation to be 97.48 F +/- 0.25 F; after the rise, the BBT was 98.09 F +/- 0.22 F. On average, he noted an increase of approximately 0.6 degrees; this corresponds with our observation that the BBT will rise from 0.4 to 0.8 degrees around the time of ovulation.

The BBT will rise 0.4 to 0.8 F near ovulation.

Note that these values are for oral temperatures; rectal or vaginal temperatures are up to one degree higher than oral temperatures. In addition, these temperatures were taken from women at rest in the early morning hours immediately upon awakening. The BBT is responsive to ovarian hormones but it is also responsive to hormones from the adrenal glands; it is lowest in the early morning hours and peaks in the late afternoon in response to the cyclic release of adrenal hormones. Thus, the above temperature ranges are only applicable to early morning BBT determinations.

The BBT should be taken in the morning upon awakening.

2. Thermometers

A common home thermometer is designed to detect and quantify the presence of a fever — an elevation of temperature above the normal, 98.6 F. Most of these thermometers are able to detect temperatures from as low as 96 F to as high as 106 F, but they are generally not precise enough to accurately detect the small temperature changes that occur during the menstrual cycle. Special thermometers for determining basal body temperatures are available at most pharmacies. They are designed to detect small changes in basal body temperature and usually measure from only 96.0 F to 100.0 F with graduated markings of 0.1 or 0.2 F. Any temperature of greater than 100.0 F would be off the scale, and, in this situation, a common home thermometer should be used to detect the height of the fever. As an alternative to the BBT thermometer, most electronic thermometers are sensitive enough to use.

We recommend that two BBT thermometers be obtained. Temperatures should be taken with both thermometers at least once per month and any differences in reading noted; therefore, if the primary thermometer is broken (not uncommon), the remainder of the cycle temperatures can be graphed with the second thermometer reading plus or minus the difference. The thermometer should be placed next to the bed in a safe place and kept away from any source of heat. It should be shaken down each night prior to falling asleep so that no vigorous activity is performed prior to the morning temperature determination.

3. Proper Use of a Thermometer

Accurate temperatures can only be obtained when the thermometer is properly inserted into the mouth, vagina, or rectum. Proper insertion includes placing the thermometer at the same depth since small variations in temperature have been noted along the vaginal and rectal canals; specifically, lower temperatures were obtained with more shallow insertions (Abrams, 1981).

> Mouth:
> The metal tip of the thermometer should be placed under the tongue with the mouth closed. Accurate determinations require at least 5 minutes, and we recommend 10 minute determinations. Do NOT drink or eat anything for at least 1 hour prior to the determination because the temperature of the mouth is easily altered by food and drink.

> Vagina:
> Many people may not initially consider the vagina as a good location for temperature determination, but it can provide excellent results. Most women assume a knee to chest position prior to insertion, and remain in this position during the entire determination. Good accuracy can be obtained after only 5 minutes of insertion. Temperatures along the vaginal canal have been found to have less variation than in the rectum; thus,

attention to the depth of insertion is less important (Abrams, 1981). The major drawback to vaginal determination is the frequent difficulty with insertion of the thermometer. Unfortunately, lubricants such as petroleum or K-Y jelly cannot be used since they may interfere with the determination of cervical mucus (this will be discussed in detail in the next section).

Rectum:

The rectum is a favored location for temperature determination in infants and small children and can provide excellent readings. As with vaginal temperatures, accurate determinations can be obtained after only 5 minutes. Insertion is most often performed in the knee to chest position, and in contrast to the vagina, any lubricant may be used. Again, there is a significant variation in temperature along the rectal canal, and attention should be paid to maintaining a constant depth of insertion; in addition, the presence of stool in the rectum may cause the temperature to appear falsely low (Abrams, 1981). In women who regularly have a bowel movement upon awakening, stool may interfere with their determinations, and one of the two other sites should be considered. Remember, passage of a bowel movement prior to determination would cause the BBT to rise from activity and defeat our purpose.

There is one safety rule during temperature determinations:

Do NOT return to sleep while the thermometer is inserted.

It will be very tempting to return to sleep, but this increases the probability of breaking the thermometer which could damage the mouth, vagina, or rectum.

4. Time of Determination

The temperature of the body normally varies across the day. It is at its lowest point in the early hours of the morning and rises slowly across the day and peaks in the afternoon. As we mentioned earlier, this cyclic change mirrors the release of hormones from the adrenal glands. Most of the time we are unaware of these rhythmic temperature changes, but, if you have ever remained awake all night, you may remember feeling very cold a few hours after midnight. This cycle is one of the ways that the body conserves energy at times when the body is less active. We have discussed the fact that any type of physical activity will generate heat and cause the body temperature to rise. However, emotions can also cause increases in temperature. To find a time in which there has been a period of inactivity and in which the likelihood of strong emotions is low, most couples determine the temperature in the early morning upon awakening.

Although early morning temperatures are theoretically the most accurate, they may be taken at other times of the day. In 1974, Zuspan and Zuspan studied the temperature charts of women who had made their determinations at different times of the day. Not surprisingly, they found that temperatures were lowest in the early morning and highest at approximately 5 PM. In addition, as long as the determinations were made at the same time each day, they were easily able to follow the chart and determine the time of ovulation. After reviewing all of the charts, they found that 5 PM and evening determinations were, on average, 0.7 F and 0.3 F above the basal determinations respectively. They contend that, if the morning determination is missed, a 5 PM or evening temperature may be graphed after corrections for times are made:

5 PM determination: Basal temp = 5 PM temp - 0.7 F

Evening determination: Basal temp = Evening - 0.3 F

In order to decrease interference, we recommend basal body temperature determinations upon awakening. However, if this is not possible, find a convenient time and determine the temperature at that time each day; try to remain calm and inactive for a short period of time prior to the determination.

The cyclical change in body temperature described above occurs in the vast majority of women. However, the body will readily adapt to a regular daily schedule. Thus, a woman who routinely works night shifts will find that her lowest basal body temperature occurs just a few hours prior to awakening in the afternoon or evening and her highest temperature occurs in the early hours of the morning. In this situation, we would determine the temperature in the afternoon or evening upon awakening.

5. Interferences

We will now discuss factors which may interfere with accurate determination of basal temperature. This information should be placed on the graph with the temperature:

   1. Any **physical activity**, however minor, will tend to increase the temperature. Thus, the thermometer should be shaken down each evening, placed next to the bed, and merely inserted into the mouth immediately after awakening. Some women find it

difficult not to move or stretch when awakening, and others have difficulty remembering to take the temperature when they awaken and realize that they have only a short amount of time to get to school, work, or other daily activities. One frequently used trick is to set the alarm for 1 or 2 hours prior to the normal time of awakening and return to sleep immediately <u>after</u> the determination.

2. **Strong emotional states** including anger or fear can increase the temperature.

3. **Illnesses** can cause fever and drastically increase the temperature.

4. Any **sleep disturbance** may alter the rhythmic change in body temperature and result in altered readings.

5.   The **environment** must be kept constant. Changes in location can cause slight but significant temperature alterations. In addition, an increase or decrease in bed covers, an electric blanket, or a heated water bed can have marked effects on temperature determinations. If necessary, make such changes between cycles.

6.   **Ingested substances** may alter temperature determinations. It is obvious that the ingestion of cold or hot liquids would have an effect on the oral temperature. However, most people fail to realize that these liquids will alter the core body temperature and influence all types of determinations. Studies have shown that the ingestion of cold liquids will lower temperatures in the vagina and, to

a lesser extent, the rectum; in addition, recent cigarette smoking will tend to increase the BBT, and erroneous values have been obtained on mornings after large amounts of alcohol have been consumed (Abrams, 1981).

7. **Medications** that you have been prescribed may affect your basal temperature. We recommend that you contact your gynecologist or the prescribing physician to find out any possible effect on your basal temperature.

6. Graphing the Results

Now, we will turn our attention to the chart at the back of this book and concentrate on the section marked Basal Body Temperature. Examine Figure 5-2 in which we have graphed a sample temperature curve. In this section of the chart, it is important to chart not only the exact temperatures but also the days of the menstrual period, interferences, and sexual intercourse:

Temperatures:

The day of the cycle is graphed horizontally across the top of this section. We have allowed up to 40 days duration for each cycle. This is much longer than the average cycle, and, if your cycle lasts longer than 40 days, your gynecologist should be consulted. The temperature scale is oriented vertically under each cycle day, and it will allow you to graph temperatures from just below 97.0 F to just above 99.0 F. Temperatures should be graphed with a dark black dot under the corresponding day of the cycle. Then, the dots can be connected to form a "temperature curve." Temperatures below 97.0 F or above 99.0 F may indicate the presence of an interfering factor or an underlying medical problem. Such high or low temperatures should be graphed by writing the exact number at the top or bottom of the graph, respectively. In Figure 5-2, the BBT was 99.4 F on cycle day 10. This was above the normal temperature range and was, therefore, written above the temperature scale. If temperatures out of this range occur frequently, please discuss these findings with your physician.

Menstrual Period:

Menstrual flow will occur at the beginning of each cycle. For each day that the bloody discharge occurs, we recommend that an X be placed over the temperature or at the top or bottom of the graph. Actually, temperature measurements are not required during this period. In Figure 5-2, the menstrual period lasted 5 days and was graphed with an X above the temperature scale.

Some women who have become pregnant will experience menstrual flow at the end of the cycle during which fertilization occurred. This flow will usually be considered light and occur for only 2 or 3 days. However, it may initially be considered to be a real menstrual period, and the woman may not realize that she has become pregnant. She will usually recognize the pregnancy during the next cycle through the initiation of morning sickness or other signs of pregnancy, and the gestational age of the baby and the expected time of delivery will be calculated from this cycle. Unfortunately, the baby will be approximately 4 weeks older than its estimated gestational age. When the time of delivery arrives, the fetus may be considered premature when it is actually a term pregnancy. For example, the fetus may have been growing in the womb for 40 weeks and be ready for delivery, but, due to misinterpreted menstrual flow, the woman may feel that the fetus is delivering prematurely at 36 weeks. Since the blood loss after fertilization is commonly small in amount or light, it may be helpful to classify the menstrual flow as light, medium, or heavy and write this vertically above the temperature dot.

Interferences:

It is very important that interfering factors be recognized. We recommend that the temperature be circled and a short description be written vertically underneath the day of the temperature determination. In Figure 5-2, the temperature dropped slightly on cycle day 7 and increased sharply between days 8 and 9. Although this occurred early in the cycle, it could, without more information, be confused with the temperature shift near ovulation. However, this woman circled the temperature on cycle day 9 to indicate that it was influenced by an interfering factor; she then provided further information by writing the word 'fever' vertically in the space below the cycle day. The temperature on cycle day 10 was even higher, requiring notation above the graph, and, it was accompanied by a cough and nasal drainage. She has accurately described the presence of an upper respiratory infection which invalidated the BBT determinations on cycle days 9 through 11. When a temperature is first obtained, the presence of an interfering factor may not be initially perceived. For example, on cycle day 9, this woman may have felt well until a high fever presented later in the day. Thus, she would need to return to the graph, circle the temperature, and write a description of the interference vertically. Notice that the occurrence of an interfering factor at the time of ovulation could obscure the true BBT shift; a chart of this type would only be useful for determining the menstrual cycle length.

Sexual Intercourse:

We recommend that a star shape be placed over the daily temperature scale when sexual intercourse occurs; alternatively, some couples prefer to chart the temperature as a star instead of a black dot. This is important for many reasons including:

1. The act of intercourse which led to fertilization can be readily identified. This will be important for calculating the length of time between insemination and ovulation which will determine the probability of conceiving a female child. Your obstetrician will also be able to use this information to determine the time at which the baby should deliver; most people refer to this date as the 'due date', but obstetricians refer to it as the EDC or Estimated Day of Confinement in the hospital.

2. Intercourse which accidentally occurs during the fertile period can be identified. It is not uncommon for the day of ovulation and the fertile period to be poorly estimated, especially during the first months of graphing the bodily changes of the menstrual cycle. If intercourse is clearly marked, a close look back at the graph will indicate accidental insemination during the fertile period.

3. An estimation of the frequency of intercourse can be obtained. This may be important if a couple were unable to conceive and subsequently consulted a fertility specialist.

7. Classical BBT Graph

Earlier, we briefly discussed Figure 5-1 in which we presented the 'Classical BBT Graph.' It represents the classic 28 day cycle with ovulation on day 14. We must stress that your BBT graph may never look like this one, but examining it will help to familiarize you with the pattern of changes reflected in ovulatory BBT graphs. Notice that, after menstruation, the temperature varies but remains just above 97.0 F. After ovulation on day 14, the temperature rises to above 98.0 F. The temperature then remains high until the next menstruation begins. There is frequently a drop in temperature just prior to the rise — it is known as the BBT nadir; this can be seen near day 14.

BBT nadir = a drop in the BBT frequently
seen just prior to the BBT shift.

Although we have depicted the pre-ovulatory (follicular phase) temperature baseline to be approximately 97.4 F and the post-ovulatory (luteal phase) temperature baseline to be approximately 98.2 F, the actual baseline temperatures will vary between women and from cycle to cycle in a given woman. The important feature is not the temperatures themselves but a lower baseline temperature prior to ovulation followed by a higher baseline temperature after ovulation.

The 'Classical BBT Graph' in Figure 5-1 depicts a very rapid or acute rise in temperature near ovulation. It is very easy in this graph to determine the day of the rise, but other graphs may not be as easily interpreted. Since it is not the absolute value of the BBT but its rise which indicates the time of ovulation, proper assignment of the BBT rise is crucial. This subject has been studied extensively by the World Health Organization (WHO), and they have defined a true shift in BBT to be one in which the transition to the phase of elevated temperature occurs in 48 hours or less and in which three consecutive daily BBTs are at least 0.2 F higher than the previous six consecutive daily temperatures (Moghissi, 1980).

In a true BBT shift, three consecutive daily temperatures are at least 0.2 F higher than the previous six consecutive daily temperatures.

Thus, an interfering factor which increases the BBT within 6 days prior to the BBT rise would cause the rise to not be considered a true rise in the BBT. The WHO must be very strict with their definition of the BBT rise because they are interested in contraception, and, with no other method of ovulation detection available, an incorrectly identified BBT rise could result in an unwanted pregnancy. If a true BBT rise is not identified in the cycle, the WHO instructs couples to continue abstinence until the next menstrual period.

Since we will be using other methods of ovulation detection concurrently, we can be more liberal in defining the BBT rise. One method taught frequently by family planning clinics is known as the 'coverline' method: a line is drawn on the graph from left to right just above the preovulatory temperatures; the point at which this 'coverline' crosses the BBT curve is considered the time of the BBT rise (Bartzen, 1967).

**The BBT rise is the point at which the
'coverline' crosses the BBT curve.**

Couples must be careful to identify and disregard temperature rises which are due to the interferences discussed earlier. Many couples who regularly use BBT graphing find that the 'coverline' is set at the same temperature in each cycle.

8. Aberrant Graphs

There will regularly be graphs which are difficult to interpret. However, their pattern may become more apparent when the day of ovulation is also indicated by changes in cervical mucus or other methods which will be described later in this book. Knowledge of the length of the luteal phase, as discussed in the Calendar Method, is also a good way to retrospectively identify ovulation in a chart which is difficult to interpret.

It is very important to be able to appreciate the lack of a temperature rise in the BBT graph. Although this may be seen in a number of women who are actually ovulating, it is suggestive, especially when found in consecutive cycles, of the absence of ovulation. These cycles commonly occur after oral contraceptive pill (OCP) use is discontinued. However, anovulatory cycles not associated with OCPs or more than two cycles without a BBT rise after cessation of OCPs should be discussed with your gynecologist. A portion of these women will require hormonal therapy, guided by their gynecologist, in order to restart regular ovulatory cycles.

9. BBT Rise and Ovulation

We have mentioned many times that the rise in BBT is associated with ovulation — this association is not disputed in medical literature. However, the exact temporal relationship and the accuracy of the method are vigorously debated. Much of the discrepancy between the available research studies stems from the fact that the exact time of ovulation is not known by the researchers; they have merely compared identifiable changes in the blood hormones such as the rise in progesterone concentration, the LH peak, or the initial rise in LH in the bloodstream. Recently, some researchers have used ultrasound to watch the developing follicle daily for evidence of ovulation. This would seem to be an ideal method of identifying the exact time of ovulation, but other researchers have performed studies which suggest that the sound waves can actually induce the follicles to rupture earlier than with the stimulation of LH alone (Testart, 1982). Thus, there is <u>no</u> perfect test for determining the exact time of ovulation; we must survey the available literature and estimate the time of occurrence of the BBT shift in relation to ovulation. Some of the more widely quoted research studies over the past years have included:

- Hilgers and Bailey in 1980: they concluded that the estimated time of ovulation was on average 0.5 days before the rise in BBT and that in 77.3% of the cycles studied the rise occurred within 2 days prior to 2 days after ovulation.
- Moghissi in 1980: this study concluded that the rise of the BBT occurs at the time of ovulation or just prior to it.
- Marinho in 1982: this study found that ovulation occurred prior to the BBT rise in 78% of their cases.

For the purposes of sex preselection, we will define the time of ovulation as 0.5 days prior to the first rise in BBT or midway between the BBT nadir (low temperature) and the first rise in BBT.

Ovulation occurs 0.5 days prior to the BBT rise.

**Ovulation occurs midway between
the BBT nadir and the BBT rise.**

Without a BBT nadir which is present in only a minority of cycles, the time of ovulation can only be identified a number of days after it has occurred. Those practicing other methods of ovulation detection will, however, be more vigilant near the time of ovulation and more able to appreciate any nadir or early temperature rise.

Example 5-1 — Determining Ovulation by BBT Graphing

Gerald and Betty are a couple who are practicing sex preselection and have been graphing Betty's basal body temperatures which can be found in Figure 5-1. The first day on which a rise in temperature is detected is day 15; thus, we estimate ovulation to have occurred 0.5 days earlier or on day 14.5. Notice that the temperature on day 15 is higher than any of the previously recorded temperatures but somewhat lower than temperatures recorded later in the cycle. Also, notice that a coverline could be placed at 97.9 F, and it would intersect the curve exactly at day 15.

Determination of the day of ovulation is more

difficult during an evolving cycle than after the cycle has been completed. Betty could, for example, attribute the temperature increase to an interfering factor rather than to ovulation. This particular cycle would have been easier to read during the cycle because a BBT nadir (low temperature) appeared on day 14 just prior to ovulation.

10. Accuracy at Predicting Ovulation

When BBT recording was first discussed in the medical literature, it was heralded as an easy and accurate method of determining ovulation. Over the past decades, many studies have found that the BBT rise can occur both a few days before or a few days after ovulation. Researchers have gradually placed less faith in the ability of BBT charting to identify ovulation. It is important to remember that we are not solely using the BBT rise to indicate ovulation but, rather, combining it with other methods to accurately identify ovulation.

Chart # ____

Female Sex Preselection Chart

CSCS Information		Present Cycle Values
ACL = Average Cycle Length = _____		MCL = Menstrual Cycle Length = _____
ALPL = Average Luteal Phase Length = _____		LPL = Luteal Phase Length= _____
ADO = Average Day of Ovulation = _____		DO = Day of Ovulation = _____

Chart # —

Female Sex Preselection Chart

CSCS Information

ACL = Average Cycle Length =

ALPL = Average Luteal Phase Length =

ADO = Average Day of Ovulation =

Present Cycle Valves

MCL = Menstrual Cycle Length =

LPL = Luteal Phase Length=

DO = Day of Ovulation =

"The secret of success is constancy to purpose."
Benjamin Disraeli

Chapter VI

Cervical Mucus Determinations

1. Introduction

One of the most visible responses of the female body to the cyclic changes in hormone production is the change in mucus secretion of the cervix. Since all women with normally cycling hormones will have a recognizable pattern of cervical mucus secretion, we were initially surprised to learn that many, if not most, women have only a rudimentary perception of these changes. Precise recognition of mucus changes can provide surprisingly accurate and inexpensive information about both the time of fertility and the time of ovulation. Therefore, we will attempt to make you comfortable with the identification and interpretation of cervical mucus changes.

2. Mucus Production and Function

First, we will review the female hormones, estrogen and progesterone, and how they affect mucus production. During the first part of the menstrual cycle, follicular cells of the ovary produce increasing amounts of estrogen, and it peaks just prior to ovulation. Estrogen is the principle hormone which affects mucus production by glands of the cervix. When estrogen is low early in the cycle, cervical mucus is scant, thick, and opaque. However, as the estrogen level rises, the rate of mucus production increases, and it becomes more fluid and clear.

**Estrogen causes cervical mucus to become
clear, slippery, and increased in volume.**

At the peak of estrogen just prior to ovulation, it is very distensible and can be stretched for many inches. This mucus has been called the Peak Symptom (**PS**) or Spinnbarkeit (**SBK**), and it is very suggestive of impending ovulation.

Peak Symptom = Spinnbarkeit $\longrightarrow$ Ovulation

After ovulation, the level of estrogen decreases and the progesterone level increases significantly; these changes cause the mucus to once again become scant, thick, and opaque.

3. General Pattern of Mucus Production

We can now discuss the changes in mucus production which occur predictably across the menstrual cycle. We will utilize an ideal 28 day cycle to illustrate these changes.

Days 1-5 : Menstrual period with shedding of the inner uterine lining formed during the previous cycle.

Days 6-7 : No or scant mucus is produced - referred to as "dry days."

Day 8 : The first evidence of mucus is found. It is usually described as sticky or tacky and is usually detectable at the vaginal opening. This mucus is opaque and white or yellow in color. When it is placed between the fingers and they are spread apart, it will not stretch but tiny peaks may be seen on the surface. This mucus may still be a barrier to sperm penetration but will soon form channels which will facilitate sperm migration past the cervix.

Days 9-12 : The mucus becomes more thin and watery and often is described as cloudy. When placed between the fingers and they are spread apart, no peaks will be seen, the surfaces will be smooth, and no stretching will be seen. This mucus is felt to be favorable to sperm and the female is generally considered to be fertile at this time. This mucus is often identified as a sensation of wetness noticed when wiping after urination.

Day 13 : The mucus becomes very profuse, slippery, clear, and stretchable in response to high estrogen levels in the virtual absence of progesterone. Many women will describe this stage as resembling raw egg white. This is Spinnbarkeit, and it will stretch several inches between two fingers. This is the time of extreme fertility and suggests that ovulation has recently, is, or will soon occur.

Day 14 : The day of ovulation. The mucus continues to be very slippery, clear, and stretchable. This is the last day upon which fertile mucus is noted; therefore, it represents the Peak Symptom.

Days 15-16 : The mucus quickly returns to sticky or tacky and then dry as estrogen levels drop slightly and progesterone levels rise.

Days 17-28 : These are considered dry days.

4. Main Objectives During Cervical Mucus Assessment

The ideal 28 day cycle is a good tool to learn the pattern of change of cervical mucus secretion; however, the vast majority of women will not have a 28 day cycle nor will they have exactly 6 days of cervical mucus formation. Since you are interested in conceiving a daughter, there is only <u>one</u> main objective upon which to concentrate while identifying and recording cervical mucus: accurately identifying the Peak Symptom.

<u>Learn to accurately identify the Peak Symptom:</u>

We will define the Peak Symptom in the same manner as Billings and Billings in 1972:

**The Peak Symptom is the last day
on which fertile mucus is noted.**

It can be a good indicator of ovulation. Studies have shown that it generally occurs within 48 hours of ovulation and may occur very close to the time of ovulation:

- Billings and Billings in 1972: they studied 22 cycles from 22 women. Their results indicated that the Peak Symptom occurred from Day -2 to Day +3 with an average of 0.9 days after ovulation.
- Hilgers and associates in 1978: they studied 74 cycles from 26 women. They found that the Peak symptom occurred from Day -2 to Day +2 in 95.4% of cycles, and it occurred, on average, 0.3 days before the estimated day of ovulation.
- Grinsted and associates in 1989: they studied 23 cycles from 21 women and found that fertile cervical mucus could usually be identified for a number of days around ovulation making determination of the exact time of ovulation difficult using this method alone. However, they did find that the absence of fertile cervical mucus was an excellent indication that ovulation was not taking place.

Example 6-1 — Determining Ovulation by the Peak Symptom

Richard and Pat are practicing sex preselection and desire a girl. Pat first noticed a wet sensation at her vagina on cycle day 8. The mucus became gradually more profuse, watery, and clear. It is now cycle day 14, and she is able to stretch the mucus for 1 to 2 inches between her fingers — this is fertile cervical mucus and the last day of its occurrence will constitute the Peak Symptom. Thus, it is near the time of ovulation and they should have intercourse to maximize their chances of conceiving a female.

5. Method of Obtaining Mucus

Another important consideration in following mucus changes is the method by which the mucus is obtained. The vast majority of women obtain mucus manually each day from the vaginal opening or from the interior of the vagina. The most common times of obtaining the mucus are at the time of basal body temperature determination, after urination, or in proximity to intercourse. A distinct and possibly superior method of inspecting the mucus involves the use of a vaginal speculum. This tool resembles the bill of a duck and is used by gynecologists to examine the vagina and cervix. Some women have found that they can use a speculum to directly assess mucus exuding from the opening of the cervix. They apply a Q-tip to the mucus and retract it; near midcycle, the mucus will stretch between the os and Q-tip corresponding to the Peak Symptom. They feel that this method is more accurate since the mucus is tested very soon after it is produced and any interference from the vaginal environment is minimized or eliminated.

There are two main reasons that cause speculums to be used only infrequently. First, the performance of this procedure is time consuming and must be done frequently near midcycle. Second, the majority of women and men do not feel comfortable with the use of a speculum. This may stem from both an unfamiliarity with the procedure and an inherent discomfort with the close anatomical inspection of themselves or their partner which may influence further sexual interaction. Despite the reservations of many people, the speculum examination is easily learned, free from significant risk of injury when performed properly, and a more accurate means of assessing cervical mucus. The use of a speculum will be discussed further in the next chapter. We recommend discussion of this subject with your gynecologist who can provide a speculum as well as interactive instruction on its proper use.

6. Description of Cervical Mucus

Describing and recording the characteristics of cervical mucus is very important. Accurate descriptions should be recorded each day in proximity to the BBT graph for comparison. The Sex Preselection Chart located at the end of this book has a section immediately below the BBT graph reserved for the description of cervical mucus. The exact words used are not important — they serve merely to help you establish the pattern of change in the mucus. However, we will encourage the use of three word descriptions; each word corresponds to a specific type of change in the mucus that is induced by estrogen. The three types of changes include: quantity, consistency, and translucency.

> 1. Estrogen alters the **QUANTITY** of mucus produced. Specifically, it increases the quantity of mucus produced. We suggest these descriptions and abbreviations:

D = none or dry
S = slight
M = moderate
A = abundant

2. Estrogen alters the **CONSISTENCY** of the mucus. It causes the mucus to become less thick and more watery. We suggest these descriptions and abbreviations:

T = thick
ST = sticky
M = moderate
SL = slippery
W = watery

3. Estrogen alters the **TRANSLUCENCY** of the mucus. Translucency describes how well light can pass through a substance. Thus, a very translucent substance might be described as clear. Estrogen causes the mucus to become more translucent (more clear). We suggest these descriptions and abbreviations:

O = opaque
C = cloudy
T = translucent or clear

In addition to the above descriptions, we recommend that the presence of Spinnbarkeit (SBK) or the Peak Symptom (PS) be recorded separately. This mucus is very abundant, slippery, and clear; it is also very elastic and has been noted to stretch a number of inches between two fingers. Again, the presence of this mucus is very suggestive of present or impending ovulation, and it should be prominently marked on your graph.

Example 6-2 — Recording Descriptions

John and Jackie are following Jackie's cervical mucus discharge and are recording their observations. Jackie has the ideal 28 day menstrual cycle. On cycle day 6, there is no mucus identified. They record:

Quantity: D = None or Dry
Consistency: Not recorded
Translucency: Not recorded

On cycle day 9, Jackie first notes a wet sensation and a small amount of mucus is obtained. They record:

Quantity: S = Slight
Consistency: T = Thick
Translucency: O = Opaque

On cycle day 14, they have watched the mucus become steadily more profuse, watery, and clear. They record:

Quantity: A = Abundant
Consistency: W = Watery
Translucency: T = Translucent or Clear

In addition, the mucus is noted to stretch inches between 2 fingers so they record the letters PS for Peak Symptom in the area marked Signs which lies just below the three descriptive boxes.

7. Interference with Accurate Determinations

The five most common interfering agents which can cause inaccurate determination of mucus characteristics are sexual activity, vaginal lubricants, feminine hygiene products, local contraceptive agents, and pharmaceuticals.

a. Recent sexual intercourse

Recent sexual intercourse is a common cause of inaccurate mucus determination. After ejaculation of seminal fluid into the female reproductive tract, a watery, cloudy discharge can be noted for up to 24 hours. This fluid most likely represents the loss of both seminal fluid in various stages of degradation and vaginal secretions. This discharge is often mistaken for fertile period mucus or, more rarely, Spinnbarkeit, and it may confound the determination of ovulation by observation of mucus changes. Therefore, we recommend that no mucus description be recorded on samples obtained within 24 hours after intercourse.

b. Vaginal lubricants

The use of vaginal lubricants during sexual intercourse may interfere with mucus determinations. Couples frequently use oil-based lubricants, such as petroleum jelly, or water-based lubricants, such as K-Y jelly to facilitate vaginal penetration during intercourse. In addition, some couples use specially prepared lotions with chemicals which stimulate the vagina. All of these, especially the lotions, should be avoided because they may cause a transient vaginal discharge which may be mistaken for fertile mucus. If initial penetration is difficult, tap water should be used to moisten both the vagina and the penis, and the initial penetrations should be very slow and gentle to allow time for vaginal muscle relaxation and the production of natural vaginal secretions.

c. Feminine hygiene products

The use of feminine hygiene products can cause inaccurate determination of cervical mucus characteristics. Allergic reaction to products such as deodorant tampons or vaginal deodorants can appear as a clear or cloudy discharge and be mistaken for fertile mucus. We discourage the use of these products and especially exposure to a new product while mucus changes are being followed closely.

d. Local contraceptive agents

The use of certain local contraceptive agents can interfere with mucus determination. The most common interferences are from spermicidal agents such as foams or jellies and from chemically treated condoms. This is an unfortunate occurrence since spermicidal agents dramatically increase the effectiveness of the barrier methods of contraception — condoms and diaphragms. Barrier methods are often employed during sex preselection attempts since it is impossible to use the more popular hormonal therapies and abstinence requires a great deal of self-control. In general, any chemical placed into the vagina is a potential source of interference, and the use of any such chemical is discouraged.

e. Pharmaceuticals

Finally, ingested pharmaceutical agents may interfere with mucus determination. For example, some antibiotics and antihistamine preparations have the side effect of changing the pattern of cervical mucus. If antibiotics are prescribed, the prescribing physician or your gynecologist should be contacted and questioned about possible interferences. Obviously, the timely and effective treatment of an infection is the most important consideration, but your physician may be able to prescribe an equally effective antibiotic that does not interfere with mucus determination. Antihistamines are found in most allergy and cold medications; we also discourage the use of these medications during mucus charting in order to decrease interference.

The most striking example of a medication which may interfere with mucus determination is the mucolytic agent guaifenesin. Mucolytic agents are drugs found in expectorant preparations which break up mucus strands. Guaifenesin is the most common expectorant ingredient in over the counter cough and cold medications; some of the more commonly prescribed agents include Hypotuss, Naldecon CX, Novahistine (DMX and Expectorant), Robitussin (A-C, CF, and PE), Triaminic Expectorant, and Tussar SF. Guaifenesin has been given to women with infertility ascribed to poor cervical mucus quality, and an improvement in the liquidity and volume of mucus was noted in some of the recipients (Lampe, 1986). Iodine containing salts are also able to soften mucus and can be found in over the counter medications including Organidin and Tussi-Organidin.

We discourage the use of expectorant medications during sex preselection because they may cause nonfertile mucus to break down and appear fertile. This may, in addition, allow sperm and other substances to pass the cervix and move higher into the female reproductive tract. The impact of this change on fertility and the infection fighting capabilities of the female tract are not fully known at this time.

*"The more we know, the more we want to know; when
we know enough, we now how much we don't know."*
Carol Orlock

Chapter VII

Cervical Observation

1. Introduction

The cervix exhibits changes during the menstrual cycle in addition to the pattern of mucus production discussed in the previous section. The cervix responds to estrogen by altering the size of its central opening (os), its texture when palpated, and its position relative to the vaginal opening.

2. Normal Anatomy

First, we will review the anatomy and function of the cervix. The term cervix actually describes the lower third of the uterus which connects the uterus with the vagina. It is a muscular tube which is more rigid than the body of the uterus, and its interior surface is lined with mucus secreting cells. The lower end of the cervix protrudes less than an inch into the vaginal cavity. When looking at the cervix from the direction of the vagina, it has the shape of a doughnut with a small hole in the middle which is named the os. It opens into the central canal of the cervix. In women who have never delivered a baby vaginally and most women who have had only Cesarean sections, the os is near perfectly round. But, in women who have had a vaginal delivery, the os will have any of a number of shapes — commonly that of a new moon.

3. Changes During the Cycle

a. Introduction

As noted above, the cervix is very responsive to the changing hormones of the menstrual cycle, and close observation will indicate cyclic changes in the size of the os, the texture of the cervix, and the position of the cervix relative to the vaginal opening. Edward F. Keefe was the first person to study and report cervical changes including positional variations and to document their usefulness as physical signs of ovulation. Since that time, many authors have recommended following cervical changes to identify ovulation.

b. Changes in os diameter

First, the rise in estrogen which occurs as ovulation approaches will cause the os to increase in diameter. Thus, as the cervical mucus glands produce slippery, watery mucus with channels for sperm to travel to the uterus, the opening to the cervix widens to further allow transport of the sperm towards an ovulated egg.

The os enlarges near ovulation.

In the vast majority of women, these diameter changes will be noticeable when the cervix is visualized, as in an examination with a speculum. In most women who have delivered a child vaginally in the past, the increase in diameter can be felt: near ovulation, a fingertip can often be inserted into the os. However, in women who have a small, circular os, the changes near midcycle may be difficult to perceive without actually looking at the os. After ovulation, the rise of progesterone and fall in estrogen will cause the os to regress to its initial small size.

c. Changes in texture

The second effect of estrogen is to change the texture of the cervix. In the early parts of the menstrual cycle, the cervix will feel rubbery and firm. For comparison, some physicians describe it as feeling like the tip of the nose. As the level of estrogen rises near ovulation, the cervix becomes softer and more pliable, and many people will favorably compare it to the lips.

The cervix becomes soft near ovulation.

After ovulation when the level of progesterone rises, the cervix will again become firm.

d. Changes in position

The third effect of estrogen is to change the position of the cervix relative to the vaginal opening. The uterus and the cervix are suspended in the pelvic cavity by strong bands of tissue called ligaments. Estrogen causes the ligaments to contract and strengthen pulling the uterus and cervix further up into the pelvic cavity. Thus, near midcycle, the uterus is further from the vaginal opening and more difficult to manually palpate.

The cervix moves higher in the vaginal canal near ovulation.

After ovulation, as the level of estrogen drops and the level of progesterone rises, the ligaments will relax and the uterus and cervix will fall closer to the vaginal opening.

e. Summary and graphing of results

We will now summarize the findings at different stages in the menstrual cycle:

Early:
  Os diameter - small or closed
  Texture - rubbery and firm
  Position - low or easily touched

Midcycle / Near ovulation:
  Os diameter - large or open
  Texture - flexible or soft
  Position - high or hard to touch

Late / After ovulation:
  Os diameter - small or closed
  Texture - rubbery and firm
  Position - low or easily touched

Example 7-1 — The Cervix Early in the Cycle

Harry and Bess are a couple who are practicing sex preselection and desire a girl. They are performing daily manual examinations of Bess' cervix to identify the time of ovulation. Just after menstruation, she is able to easily find her cervix which feels firm with some flexibility — not unlike the pliability of the tip of her nose. She is able to find her os, but it is small and unable to accept the tip of her finger. Thus, she is in the early or infertile period of the cycle.

Example 7-2 — The Cervix Near Midcycle

Harry and Bess continue to follow cervical changes during the menstrual cycle. She has an ideal menstrual cycle. Near day 14, she notices that the cervix has become progressively more difficult to touch and that it is now high up in the vaginal canal. In addition, it has become more soft, and the os has become open to the point that the tip of the finger can be inserted. These changes are indicative of impending ovulation. Harry and Bess will now be watching the other methods of ovulation determination very closely to estimate the exact day of ovulation as accurately as possible. Since they desire a female child they will have intercourse as close to the time of ovulation as possible.

4. Recording Cervical Changes

The information obtained from examination of the cervix should be recorded with the basal body temperature graph and mucus determinations. This will readily allow the use of all of the information to estimate the day of ovulation. We recommend the following designations for the simplification of charting:

Os diameter:
   S = Small
   I = Intermediate
   L = Large

Texture:
   F = Firm
   I = Intermediate
   S = Soft

Position:
   L = Low
   I = Intermediate
   H = High

5. Changes with Pregnancy

The cervix may also give indications that the female partner is pregnant. Since couples who have been examining the cervix may knowingly or unknowingly continue to examine the cervix after conception, they may encounter the main cervical sign of pregnancy:

> **Chadwick's sign** - the cervix becomes larger, much softer, and develops a bluish discoloration due to the increase in blood supply.

This sign first presents many weeks after conception. Therefore, couples should have already noted many other indications of pregnancy such as the absence of menstruation and the absence of a fall in basal body temperature after the fertilization.

6. Methods of Examining the Cervix

a. Manual examination

Examination of the cervix is not difficult but requires persistence and patience. The vast majority of people examine the cervix manually — with their hands alone. This type of examination requires no more internal manipulation than the checking of a diaphragm. In addition, as long as the introduced hand is clean and the fingernails are well trimmed, there is very little risk of infection or bleeding due to laceration of the vaginal walls. The steps to be followed in examining the cervix include:

> 1. <u>The examination should occur at the same time each day.</u> There are slight changes in cervical position and texture during the course of each day which may interfere with your determinations. An optimal time for such examinations has not been

established, and most couples merely include this examination with their BBT and mucus determinations.

2. <u>The examining hands should be cleaned thoroughly with an antibacterial soap.</u>

3. <u>Do **NOT** use a lubrication substance for the examining fingers.</u> People are often tempted to use petroleum or K-Y (water-based) jelly on the fingers when the vaginal opening is dry and the fingers are difficult to insert. This practice will, however, preclude any examination of the cervical mucus wasting a valuable source of information. If entering the vagina is difficult, the fingers should be made wet with tap water. The requirement of some type of lubrication is often an indication of the infertile period.

4. <u>The most accurate determinations of cervical position occur when both the bladder and rectum are empty.</u> The bladder lies directly in front of the vaginal canal while the rectum lies behind it. Pressure exerted by the contents of either cavity can cause the cervix to change position.

5. <u>The subject should be in the same position for each examination.</u> This requirement is a direct result of the effect of gravity on the uterus. In the vertical position, gravity will draw the cervix further into the vaginal canal and, thus, closer to the introitus.

   Each examination of the cervix may be performed in either the vertical or horizontal position. For self examinations, the vertical position is often preferred because the action of gravity will make the cervix easier to palpate. The subject should stand with one leg elevated slightly above the other by resting it on an object such as the side of a bed or a toilet seat. The fingers of one hand are then inserted carefully into the vagina and moved toward the head. This insertion of fingers should mimic the insertion of a tampon. If the cervix is not readily palpable, gentle pressure can be applied to the abdomen just below the navel. This places pressure on the uterus and forces the cervix closer to the vaginal opening. After the cervix is identified, the pressure should be released since it would interfere with determination of the natural cervical position.

The horizontal position is most often used by couples when the male partner is performing the daily exams. The subject lies on her back with her thighs moved apart; the examination then proceeds as described above. Couples may want to use the vertical position when the partner finds the cervix difficult to locate or assess when in the horizontal position.

6. <u>The examinations should be performed daily</u>. During each exam, the os diameter, cervix texture, and cervical position should be assessed. In addition, most participants simultaneously assess the characteristics of the cervical mucus as outlined in the previous chapter.

7. <u>The hands should be cleaned thoroughly with antibacterial soap at the end of each determination.</u>

Although manual inspection of the cervix is a good method during sex preselection, **it should not be used during pregnancy:** the developing fetus is very susceptible to infections, and even the low incidence of infection with manual inspection is not acceptable. In addition, palpation during the later months of pregnancy can induce labor. It may be tempting to examine the cervix during pregnancy once the techniques have been practiced, but we strongly advise against it.

b. Use of a speculum

A more objective way of determining cervical changes is through the use of a speculum. This is the viewing instrument used by physicians to adequately assess the vagina and cervix. It is shaped like the bill of a duck and made of either metal or strong plastic. They are reusable when properly cleansed both before and after each use. A speculum may be used either by a solitary female when a mirror and a light source are used or by a couple with the male partner assessing the cervical changes. The steps associated with using a speculum would include:

1. <u>Clean the speculum thoroughly.</u>

2. <u>The subject should lie on her back with her knees bent and thighs moved apart as far as possible.</u>

3. <u>A light source should be aimed at the vaginal canal,</u> and, if self-inspection is being performed, <u>a mirror should be placed to adequately view the area.</u>

4. <u>A finger of the partner or the subject's non-dominant hand is inserted in the vagina,</u> and it exerts a gentle pressure down toward the rectum.

5. <u>Insert the closed speculum into the vagina over the inserted finger with the handle pointing toward one of the thighs.</u> As it is advanced, rotate the handle down to the anus.

6. <u>If the speculum is not readily insertable, wet it with water.</u> We discourage the use of petroleum or water-based lubricants as, again, this may interfere with the determination of cervical mucus characteristics.

7. <u>Open the speculum by pressing the handles together and view the cervix.</u> Most of the specula can be held in the open position by the use of a threaded bolt and nut built onto their side regions.

8. <u>Identify the os diameter, the texture of the cervix, and the cervical position.</u> In addition, note the amount of cervical mucus at the os and obtain a sample for inspection. At this time, some couples identify Spinnbarkeit by touching a Q-tip to the os and retracting it — true Spinnbarkeit mucus will stretch between the Q-tip and os for inches.

9. <u>Carefully close the speculum without trapping the walls of the vagina.</u> Pull it out gently while rotating the handle towards a thigh.

10. <u>Clean the speculum thoroughly.</u>

This examination should be short, painless, and safe. A speculum can be obtained from a medical supply house or your gynecologist. We strongly encourage you to discuss this procedure with your gynecologist before attempting it at home; he or she can interactively answer your questions and provide further instruction on the safe use of a speculum

"Curiouser and curiouser."
Lewis Carroll

Chapter VIII

Mittleschmerz

Another indicator of ovulation is Mittleschmerz which has been defined in Taber's Cyclopedic Medical Dictionary (1981) as:

> *"Abdominal pain midway between menstrual periods, occurring at the time of ovulation and from the ovulation site."*

Although only a small percentage of women — approximately 25% (Cunningham, 1993) — perceive this pain, it is very specific for ovulation. The pain is characteristically located in the right or left lower abdomen, but its quality and duration are very variable. Descriptions of the quality range from sharp to dull, and descriptions of the duration range from seconds to hours. However, the most common presentation is a short, sharp pain, and the pain characteristics are often constant from cycle to cycle in a given woman.

1. The Origin of Mittleschmerz

For many years, physicians have concluded that the pain of Mittleschmerz arises when the egg punctures the capsule around the ovary at the time of ovulation; this can be considered the classical explanation. To better understand this theory, we can review the changes in the ovary as ovulation approaches. As the egg and developing follicular cells respond to follicle stimulating hormone (FSH), the cells multiply and secrete fluid making the follicle larger. This enlarging follicle moves to the outer edge of the ovary and stretches the covering of the ovary which is connected to nerves. Most of the organs in the abdominal region are covered by a tissue which is connected to nerves which can convey pain messages. For example, when the appendix becomes inflamed in appendicitis, its outer covering is stretched and a poorly localized abdominal pain is felt. Similarly, at midcycle, the outer covering of the ovary is punctured at ovulation as the egg is expelled toward the fallopian tubes, and the pain of Mittleschmerz is felt. Differences in the number of nerves to the covering of the ovary may explain the fact that only a small number of women recognize the pain. Fortunately, a larger number of women may perceive the pain when actively watching for it near the time of ovulation.

Although the above theory is still upheld by many physicians today, others feel that the pain is instead caused by contraction of muscles in the female tract (O'Hearlihy, 1980) or by irritation of the abdominal walls by fluid released near the time of ovulation.

2. Bounce Test

Dr. Howard I. Shapiro in "The Birth Control Book (1978)" described an interesting method for increasing the perception of ovulatory pain called the "Bounce Test." He recommended moving to a sitting position abruptly three to four times each morning and evening, beginning six days prior to expected ovulation. He contends that these Bounce Tests will allow up to one-third of women to perceive ovulatory pain.

3. Location of Mittleschmerz

The pain is felt randomly in either the left or right lower abdomen. We must remember that ovulation does not alternate between sides each month. Since ovulation occurs on the right or left randomly, Mittleschmerz is felt in a similar fashion. Although it may alternate from side to side, it will frequently be felt on the same side in consecutive cycles.

4. Relationship of Mittleschmerz to Ovulation

Although the classical understanding of Mittleschmerz suggests that the pain will be felt exactly at the time of ovulation, recent studies of ovulation have challenged this assumption:

> - O'Hearlihy and colleagues in 1980 studied 96 women and determined the time of ovulation with ultrasound examinations. Mittleschmerz was identified in 34 women (35%), and, in the 27 women in which the pain was localized to the left or right, it corresponded with the side of follicle enlargement. The pain did not last more than 24 hours in any of the women, and in 31 (91%), it occurred 24 to 48 hours prior to ovulation. They attributed the pain to contraction of muscles within the ovary.
> - Grinsted and colleagues in 1989 studied 21 previously infertile women and found 6 (29%) to have Mittleschmerz. Although this is a very small number of patients, they found that the pain occurred before ovulation in 4 patients, both before and after ovulation in one patient, and after ovulation in one patient. They concluded that it is not a reliable indicator of ovulation. In contrast, we feel that they did not have a large enough number of patients to draw such a conclusion.

For the purposes of sex preselection, we will designate the pain of Mittleschmerz to occur in the interval 24 to 48 hours prior to ovulation.

Mittleschmerz occurs 24 to 48 hours prior to ovulation.

Example 8-1 — Mittleschmerz and Ovulation

Franklin and Eleanor are practicing sex preselection and desire a girl. Eleanor has long noted a sharp pain in the lower right or left abdomen (or pelvic region) in between menstrual cycles. They practice all of the methods described previously in order to accurately follow changes in her menstrual cycle. They begin to recognize the fertile period by the date on the calendar, the production of more fertile mucus, and changes in the cervix. At that time, Eleanor begins to concentrate on identifying the abdominal pain that she has felt in the past. Since Franklin and Eleanor desire a girl and Mittleschmerz occurs 24 to 48 hours before the time of ovulation, they begin to have intercourse one day after the pain has been identified.

Example 8-2 — Bounce Pain and Ovulation

Herbert and Lou are a couple practicing sex preselection and desire a daughter. Lou had never noticed a consistent abdominal pain near midcycle prior to practicing sex selection, and during her first cycle, no pain was perceived. They were practicing all of the methods described in the previous chapters and began to use the Bounce Method to attempt to identify Mittleschmerz. At the beginning of the fertile period, she began to stand in front of a chair and move abruptly to a sitting position three times each morning before leaving for work and three times each evening upon return from work. During successive cycles, she noted a sharp abdominal pain in the lower left or right abdomen (or pelvic region) that was noted only when she moved abruptly into a sitting position near the expected time ovulation. Since Herbert and Lou desire a girl, they will plan to have intercourse 24 to 48 hours after the next occurrence of the Bounce pain. Ovulation should occur within 24 to 48 hours of this pain.

5. Graphing Ovulatory Pain

We recommend noting the presence of Mittleschmerz or Bounce pain on the BBT graph below the daily temperature reading with a single letter:

M = Mittleschmerz
B = Bounce

On each day that Mittleschmerz is actively sought or a Bounce Test is performed, some notation should be made on the chart; we recommend that a 0 be placed in the assigned box. This will be important if ovulation is estimated poorly.

Example 8-3 — Improper Timing of Bounce Pain Tests

Calvin and Grace are a couple who have been practicing sex preselection with the hope of having a girl. Grace noticed Bounce pain in the two previous cycles just prior to the estimated time of ovulation as judged by other methods, and they plan to use this pain as their primary indicator of ovulation in the upcoming cycle. She has had ideal cycles in the past, and, therefore, they perform Bounce Tests on cycle days 12 through 16 without any pain noted. They chart a 0 in the Mittleschmerz blank underneath each of the days. At the end of the cycle, other indicators of ovulation suggest that ovulation occurred on cycle day 20; they attribute the lengthened follicular phase to emotional stress she felt with the death of a relative which occurred just after menstruation. Since they charted a 0 on each day that the Bounce Test was performed, they know that the test was merely performed at the wrong time. If no mark had been placed on the chart, they might have mistakenly concluded that no Bounce pain was present during the cycle.

6. Interfering Abdominal Pains

Mittleschmerz is a very nonspecific pain which can be imitated by many other abdominal conditions including:

> Viral infections of the bowels (viral gastroenteritis)
> Constipation
> Lower abdominal muscle strains
> Urinary tract infections (UTIs)
> Complications of sexually transmitted diseases (STDs)
> Bacterial infections of the bowels
> Appendicitis
> Ovarian cysts or other abnormalities
> Pregnancies outside of the uterus (ectopic)

Although the presence of this pain can be a good method for determining the time of ovulation, it should not be used alone.

Do NOT use Mittleschmerz alone to determine ovulation.

When used without other methods of ovulation detection, the interfering pains can easily be mistaken for the true pain of ovulation.

Example 8-4 — Abdominal Pains Interfering with Mittleschmerz

Warren and Florence are a couple who are practicing sex preselection and desire a girl. When they first began to examine each of her menstrual cycles, they used many methods to determine the exact time of ovulation. However, since she had regular cycles and a lower abdominal pain preceding ovulation by 24 hours in each cycle, they decided to cease following all of the methods except Mittleschmerz and to have intercourse 24 hours after the pain was first noted. On cycle day 16, she began to feel a dull ache in her lower left abdomen, and they had intercourse on day 17. Later on day 17, however, the pain intensified and she began to have diarrhea. Realizing that they may have had intercourse at an improper time they began to look for other signs of ovulation. All the methods pointed to cycle day 21 as the time of ovulation, and they had intercourse on Day -4 relative to ovulation. Although they desire a girl, they have had intercourse on a day which would produce fewer (approximately 40%) females. Fortunately, Florence did not become pregnant on that cycle, and, in future cycles, they used many methods to determine the time of ovulation.

"Babies are such a nice way to start people."
                    Don Herold

Chapter IX

Cervical Chemistry

The chemistry of cervical mucus changes with the menstrual cycle. The most important change for sex preselection is that the glucose content of cervical mucus increases as ovulation approaches.

Cervical mucus contains more glucose near ovulation.

This increase in glucose was first recognized and studied by Birnberg and colleagues in 1958. They placed short strips of a paper impregnated with chemicals known as Tes-Tape® into the cervical canal near the time of ovulation. This paper indicates the glucose content of its environment by changing color. These mucus glucose tests were performed on ovulating women who were about to undergo surgical removal of the uterus (hysterectomy); they would test the mucus, perform the surgery, and then examine the ovaries to identify the proximity to ovulation. Birnberg found that, at approximately 2 days prior to their estimated day of ovulation, a faint color change could be detected in the Tes-Tape® strip reflecting a low glucose concentration. The color then reached its maximal intensity on the day of ovulation; this was confirmed by finding recently ruptured follicles after the glucose reagent paper had revealed a very intense color. The paper would gradually return to its original color over the first 2 or 3 days after ovulation. Thus, Birnberg concluded that the glucose content of cervical mucus increases near ovulation and that changes in Tes-Tape® color could reliably indicate this change in glucose content.

2. Tes-Tape®

Tes-Tape®, also known as Glucose Enzymatic Test Strip, was developed in 1956 by Dr. A. S. Keston and has been used for almost 40 years to test urine samples for the presence of glucose. It is a thin roll of paper in a plastic container, and each roll will allow for approximately 100 determinations. When the test strip comes in contact with glucose, chemical reactions occur which result in a change in its color. Higher concentrations of glucose will cause a more significant color change; it is yellow when initially purchased, will turn green, and then eventually turn blue as the glucose concentration increases.

Tes-Tape® steadily turns to green and then blue as the glucose content of cervical mucus increases.

Thus, at ovulation, the color should approach dark blue.

Tes-Tape® has been found to be both sensitive and accurate at identifying glucose in urine samples: studies have found that a color change will be found with glucose concentrations of 0.05% or more and that urine glucose determinations are accurate 96% of the time (Duffy, 1992). Obviously, we will be testing cervical mucus instead of urine, but we should obtain reliable results with the use of glucose test strips.

3. Testing Cervical Mucus

The following should be considered when testing mucus:

a. Storage

The plastic container of paper should be kept in a place removed from strong sources of light, high humidity, or the extremes of heat. Tes-Tape® which becomes dark yellow or yellowish-brown may be damaged and should be discarded. Paper tape in which no color change has been noted or in which damage has been suspected can be tested by exposure to a glucose containing solution. Any nationally known beverage which contains sugar can be used for this test. It should be freshly opened and exposed to the paper which should quickly turn to a deep blue color. Remember, the beverage must contain sugar for this test to be successful. Most diet beverages contain the artificial sweetener aspartame (NutraSweet®, the NutraSweet Co.) instead of sugar and will not affect the color of the paper.

After the plastic wrapper is removed, the paper should be used within 4 months or discarded. We recommend replacement of the paper after every 4 menstrual cycles. It may be helpful to test a small number of mucus samples with both the new and old rolls to identify any slight differences in coloration. This practice is analogous to the simultaneous use of two BBT thermometers.

b. Applying cervical mucus

The glucose test paper should be placed on a clean, dry surface. Then, a small amount of mucus should be obtained, as discussed in the chapter on mucus determination, and applied to the paper. A color change to deep green or deep blue, due to high glucose concentrations in the mucus, usually occurs within 5 minutes, but Birnberg found that the first evidence of color change (a pale green color) appeared from 3 to 30 minutes after exposure to the mucus. Thus, early determinations which initially appear negative should be followed for up to 30 minutes to confirm that a pale green color does not develop.

A more direct method of testing cervical mucus can be accomplished through the use of a vaginal speculum. As we described earlier, in Chapter VII, the speculum can allow direct visualization of the cervix. The paper can then be held by a freshly washed or gloved hand and applied to the mucus emanating from the cervical os. This reduces any interference from the vaginal environment, and, thus, it may allow earlier determination of the initial increase in glucose content and more reliable determination of the glucose peak.

c. Interferences

The most common cause of a falsely positive cervical mucus glucose test is exposure to another source of glucose. Body fluids including tears, saliva, or perspiration contain enough glucose to influence a test. Thus, we recommend that the paper tape only be touched by a freshly washed or gloved hand. In addition, the chlorine residues from cleansing agents which may be present near lavatories may cause the paper tape to test positive without exposure to glucose. Thus, the tape should only be placed on clean, dry surfaces which are free from chlorine residues.

4. Charting the Results

The results from cervical mucus testing should be charted along with any information obtained from other methods. There are two methods which are commonly used to report changes in the color of test paper: the color chart and descriptive methods.

a. Color chart method

Each roll of paper tape is accompanied by a color chart to which the paper can be compared after the determination. There are 5 pictures on the color chart which range from yellow to blue and are labelled from 0 to ++++. Each color corresponds to a specific glucose concentration from 0 to 2%. Since the use of multiple plus signs would consume a great deal of space on the chart, we recommend the following notations:

$$
\begin{aligned}
0 &= 0 &&= 0 \\
1 &= + &&= 0.10\% \\
2 &= ++ &&= 0.25\% \\
3 &= +++ &&= 0.5\% \\
4 &= ++++ &&= 2.0\%
\end{aligned}
$$

Many couples prefer this method because the test paper can merely be compared to the color chart and the proper number recorded without a great deal of thought.

b. Descriptive method

Another method of charting the color changes is called the descriptive method. The test paper is closely inspected and mentally assigned a specific color on the spectrum from yellow to blue. We recommend the following short notations as descriptions of the color change:

$$\begin{aligned}
\mathbf{Y} &= \text{Yellow} \\
\mathbf{YG} &= \text{Yellow - Green} \\
\mathbf{G} &= \text{Green} \\
\mathbf{BG} &= \text{Blue - Green} \\
\mathbf{B} &= \text{Blue — possible} \\
\mathbf{DB} &= \text{Dark Blue — probable ovulation}
\end{aligned}$$

5. Identification of Ovulation

Accurate identification of the time of ovulation is very important for you since you desire a female child. It is important to understand that the glucose in cervical mucus peaks near ovulation but does not necessarily reach the concentration of 2% glucose required to turn the test paper a dark blue color. Most women will produce a dark blue test near ovulation, but women who do not produce a dark blue test paper should consider the presence of the darkest color to coincide with ovulation.

Example 9-1 — Cervical Mucus Chemistry and Ovulation

Woodrow and Edith are a couple practicing sex preselection who desire a girl. They have been following changes in Edith's cervical mucus glucose concentration using Tes-Tape® and found that no dark blue color was ever noted. However, a blue-green color was consistently noted, and the first day of its appearance corresponded well with other indicators of ovulation. Since they desire a female child, they will plan to have intercourse in the next cycle on the first day in which the blue-green color is noted.

From this example, we can again see that the absolute concentration of glucose is not important — Edith's secretions never had a glucose concentration which registered more than blue-green on the test paper. We should focus, instead, on the pattern of glucose change because ovulation is associated with the peak in glucose concentration.

7. Alternative Products

Although Tes-Tape® has been widely available for decades, it may not be present in a particular pharmacy. In this situation, we would recommend the use of Clinistix® reagent strips. These strips are also widely available, used by diabetics to test urine for glucose, and able to detect glucose concentrations as low as 0.10%. Each reagent strip has only a small square at one end which changes color when contacted by glucose; therefore, they may be more difficult to use than Tes-Tape®.

Tes-Tape® is a registered trademark of Eli Lilly and Company, Lilly Corporate Center, Indianapolis, IN, 46285
Clinistix® is a registered trademark of Miles, Inc., Diagnostics Division, Elkhart, IN, 46515

> *"Sugar and spice and everything nice,*
>   *that's what little girls are made of."*
> *"Snips and snails and puppy dog tails,*
>   *that's what little boys are made of.*
>   **Nursery rhyme**

Chapter X
Urine LH Testing

An excellent new method for estimating the time of ovulation is the determination of luteinizing hormone, or LH, in the urine.

1. Review of Hormonal Changes

Throughout the first half of the cycle, cells of the ovarian follicle stimulated by FSH produce increasing levels of estrogen. When the estrogen level becomes very high, the pituitary gland of the brain decreases production of FSH and begins to rapidly produce LH. This LH surge most often begins early in the morning, and the blood level rises over the next several hours (Seikel et al, 1982). It stimulates the follicle to rupture with ovulation of the egg, and it induces most of the follicle cells to change to the production of progesterone. Once in the blood stream, LH is readily excreted into the urine, and urine levels also peak prior to ovulation.

2. Relationship of Urine LH and Ovulation

Studies have correlated the first positive urine LH test with ovulation. The first positive test has always been found to occur prior to ovulation, but the time interval between them has become shorter as initial studies have been repeated over the past decade. Recently, Martinez and associates in 1991 found that the first positive test occurred between 16 and 28 hours before ovulation; their findings correlated well with other recent research studies (Singh et al, 1984; Vermesh et al, 1987). For the purposes of sex preselection, we will consider the first positive urine LH test to occur just less than one day prior to ovulation.

The first positive urine LH test occurs approximately one day before ovulation.

3. Urine LH Tests

There are now a large variety of urine LH tests available, without a prescription, at local pharmacies. In each test, a small amount of urine is treated with specially prepared solutions. If even a small quantity of LH is present in the urine, a color change will occur, and the test is considered positive. The test kits usually allow between 5 and 10 determinations of urine LH and cost approximately $25 to $50 per kit — $5 per test. All of the test kits report very high accuracy rates (just below 100%). The following points should be considered when testing urine:

a. Number of daily determinations

Urine determinations can be made once per day with an evening urine or twice per day with both the first morning urine and an evening urine. We recommend twice daily determinations because at least one study using 2 determinations found that only one positive test occurred in approximately one-quarter of cycles (Martinez et al, 1991). Thus, testing once per day may miss the LH peak in a significant number of cycles. Unfortunately, this is twice as expensive which may be prohibitive. In all evening determinations, voiding should not have occurred within 4 hours of obtaining the evening urine.

b. Time of determination

If only one daily determination is made, what is the best time? Most of the information supplied with the urine test kits state that the best time to test the urine is just after awakening in the morning. This is consistent with common sense because, at this time, the urine is concentrated and the level of LH may be higher. However, a recent study found that evening urine tests more reliably predicted ovulation (Luciano et al, 1990). This finding can be easily explained. As we have noted, the blood LH surge usually begins in the morning hours. Consequently, an AM urine test may not identify the rise because a sufficient amount of LH has not been filtered out of the blood by the kidneys; the evening urine will, however, have a positive test. Thus, we recommend that single daily urine tests be performed on evening urine samples.

c. Number of days of determination

We recommend that testing begin at least 5 to 6 days prior to the expected time of ovulation. This substantially increases the cost of urine testing, but it also will allow time for errors in estimation of ovulation. Alternatively, couples may begin determinations when they first identify the fertile period such as at the first sign of fertile cervical mucus.

d. Absence of positive tests

If no LH surge is detected by the expected time of ovulation, testing should be continued. Inaccurate estimation of ovulation is more common, in our experience, than either the absence of ovulation or a missed LH peak. If no LH surge continues to be detected and other changes of ovulation are not observed, ovulation might not have occurred during that cycle.

If a cycle without ovulation is suspected, your charts and test information should be reviewed with your gynecologist. It is important to remember that the action of oral contraceptive pills is to suppress ovulation, and it is not uncommon to have cycles without ovulation in the first few months after discontinuation of the pills.

e. First positive urine test

In the studies of urine LH test kits, the time of ovulation has been correlated with the first positive urine test. We can only be sure that we have witnessed the first positive urine test if we have tested the urine previously and found it to be negative. When the first urine test that we perform in a given month has a positive result, we do not know whether ovulation will follow, is occurring, or has already passed. In this situation, we would either discard this method and follow other indicators of ovulation or wait until the next cycle and begin the urine tests at an earlier time.

The presence of only one or two negative tests prior to the first positive test should cause the couple to consider beginning testing earlier in the next cycle. Conversely, a long string of negative results prior to the first positive test should help the couple to feel comfortable with beginning the testing at a later date in the next cycle.

f. Discontinuing testing

After the first positive urine LH test, no further testing is required because ovulation has been correlated only with the first positive test and the urine tests will usually continue to be positive. In a study which performed tests twice daily, positive results were obtained up to 5 consecutive times, but, on average, two positive tests occurred (Martinez et al, 1991).

Some couples will want to immediately repeat any first positive test on a urine sample to make sure that the test is not falsely positive. In addition, any test in which there is a question about the result, such as a partial color change, should be repeated as soon as possible.

g. Interferences

There are a number of situations such as a recent or present pregnancy which may interfere with testing. In addition, certain medications, in particular fertility drugs, may interfere with these tests. Your gynecologist should be contacted with any questions regarding possible interference.

Example 10-1 — Urine LH Tests and Ovulation

Theodore and Alice are a couple who are practicing sex preselection and desire a girl. They are following all of the methods previously described and have found her cervical mucus production to begin on average 5 days prior to ovulation. Beginning after she first notes fertile mucus production, she begins to test each evening urine with an LH test kit. She notes the first positive test a few days later on the evening of day 13. Thus, we would expect ovulation to occur somewhere between the morning and evening of day 14 — 16 to 28 hours after the first positive test. Since Theodore and Alice desire a girl, they would have intercourse on day 14; they can have multiple acts of intercourse on day 14 but should cease before day 15.

We have purposefully discussed this method of ovulation determination near the end of this book. It is both a simple and accurate method of determining ovulation, and we have found that most couples will tend to focus on the urine LH test to the exclusion of the other more time consuming and subjective methods of determining ovulation. Overreliance on these tests has two major disadvantages. First, despite the presence of ovulation in a given cycle, a positive urine test may not be obtained; this is especially common when the urine is tested only once daily. More importantly, however, a positive result may falsely occur earlier or later in the cycle and result in insemination at a time that predisposes to the conception of male offspring; close observation of the other indicators of ovulation should yield information which readily conflicts with the falsely positive result and prevents insemination at the wrong time.

4. Graphing the Results

The results of each urine LH test should be included on the Sex Preselection Chart at the back of this book. The space reserved for recording these results is divided by a forward slash (/); morning and evening test results should be written above and below the line respectively. A negative urine LH test should be graphed simply with a (-) above or below the slash under the appropriate day on the BBT graph. Similarly, each positive test should be noted with a (+) under the appropriate day. Again, no more testing is required after the first positive test, and extra tests may be saved for the next month, if needed.

Chapter XI

Integrating the Methods

Now that we have discussed each different method of observing the menstrual cycle, we will integrate the information that they yield to identify the four major phases of the menstrual cycle: the days prior to the fertile period, the days of the fertile period, the day of ovulation, and the days after ovulation.

1. Before the Fertile Period

First, we will identify the days prior to the fertile period. This will include the days of menstrual flow and the following days during which the probability of conception is low. At this time, the methods yield the following information:

   - a low BBT
   - dry mucus
   - a low, firm cervix with a closed os
   - yellow glucose test paper
   - a (-) urinary LH determination

2. Fertile Period

   We will, next, identify the fertile period which includes the days prior to ovulation in which the probability of conception is increasing. This can be estimated to begin up to 6 days prior to ovulation, and the methods give the following information:

- low BBT
- progressively increased mucus production
- cervix moving from low to high
- cervical os progressively opening
- initially (-) then (+) Mittleschmerz/Bounce pain
- glucose test paper turning first green and then more blue
- initially (-) and then (+) urinary LH determination

These first two phases correspond to the follicular phase described in Chapter II.

3. Ovulation

We will then identify the day of ovulation. This is a discrete event, and, thus, it is by far the shortest of the phases. We have found that precise identification of this phase is especially difficult in the first few cycles but becomes progressively easier with subsequent cycles. Accurate detection of ovulation is the foundation of female preselection. The methods indicate:

- a low BBT - just prior to the rise
- profuse clear mucus and then Spinnbarkeit
- a high, soft cervix with an open os
- resolving Mittleschmerz/Bounce pain
- blue or dark blue glucose test paper
- urinary LH determinations (+)

4. After Ovulation

Finally, we will identify the days after ovulation which include the few days of high probability of conception which occur immediately after ovulation and the remainder of the cycle in which the probability of conception is low. This period corresponds to the luteal phase described in Chapter II:

- a high BBT
- transiently fertile but regressing to dry mucus
- a low, firm cervix with a closed os
- initially lighter green then yellow glucose test paper
- urinary LH determinations (-)

Notice that each phase is not determined by one specific method but by a constellation of findings from many different methods. This prevents incorrect information from one of the methods from causing us to inaccurately estimate the early fertile period or the time of ovulation. These phases should be identified during each menstrual cycle. In the final analysis, the determination of each phase is educated guessing, and, as more information is collected through close observation of the menstrual cycle, your estimations will become more reliable — your guesses will become more educated.

"The whole is different from the sum of its parts."
A Principle of Gestalt Psychology

Chapter XII

Female Sex Preselection

*"Luck is what happens when
preparation meets opportunity."*
Branch Rickey

The key to maximizing the conception of females is accurate
determination of the time of ovulation. **All** of the methods which
we have discussed can be useful in determining ovulation. We
have further evaluated the methods as excellent, good, fair or
unknown depending upon our impression of their usefulness for
identifying the time of ovulation.

Excellent Methods:

Methods have been classified as excellent if:
1. They provide information very close to the time
of ovulation
2. They are applicable to the majority of women
3. They provide results which are easy to identify
and interpret.

Urine LH Testing - this is the **only** method which we consider
excellent. It provides information very close to the time of
ovulation: recent studies have found the urine LH rise to precede
ovulation by 16 to 28 hours (Martinez et al, 1991). Thus, the
optimal time for female preselection occurs just less than 1 day
after the first positive urine LH test. The tests can be performed

by all women, although many couples may not be able to afford the expense which is approximately $5 per determination. A positive test result is easily identified, and most test kits report an accuracy that approaches 100%.

Good Methods:

Methods have been classified as good if:
1. They are good at estimating the time of ovulation
2. They can be mastered by the majority of women with only moderate time or expense.

Cervical Mucus Changes - recent studies have revealed a good correlation between the Peak Symptom and the time of ovulation, and it can be used by the majority of women without significant expense. However, this method is not considered excellent because accurate mucus determinations require a significant amount of practice. For the purpose of sex preselection, we estimate ovulation to occur exactly at the time of the Peak Symptom — the last day of fertile cervical mucus production. Thus, to increase the probability of a female child, intercourse should occur at the time of the Peak symptom.

Cervical Changes - this method is also not considered excellent because accurate assessment of changes requires practice and a significant allotment of time. For female preselection, insemination should occur at the time when the cervix is soft and difficult to palpate, and when the os is open and readily distensible. Alone, this method would be difficult for the even the ardent observer, but it can be quite helpful for identifying the time of ovulation when combined with mucus determinations.

BBT Graphing - this method usually provides information within 48 hours of the time of ovulation. It does not approach the accuracy of LH testing, but it is certainly useful when practiced in conjunction with other methods. We estimate that ovulation occurs 0.5 days prior to the first BBT rise or midway between the BBT nadir and the first BBT rise. This method is truly applicable to the majority of women since the recording of temperature is easily performed, understood, and afforded. The exact occurrence of the temperature rise may be difficult to ascertain, and this first day of rise may have the highest probability of conception of females. However, an increased incidence of female offspring has also been noted on the day before and the day after the temperature rise (Guerrero, 1974).

Notice that BBT graphing complements urine LH testing well. Urine testing gives information about the beginning of the female days while BBT graphing gives information about the end of the female days. To maximize conception of female offspring, acts of intercourse can commence shortly after the first positive urine LH test and continue until the first evidence of the BBT rise (Day +1) — this period of female preselection should last approximately 48 hours.

Fair Methods:

Methods have been classified as fair if:
1. They roughly approximate the time of ovulation
2. They are present in only a minority of women
3. Their characteristic signs are more difficult to distinguish.

Calendar Method - this is considered only a fair method of determining ovulation because it can help to determine the time of ovulation when looking back at a cycle, but it provides only a rough approximation of the time of ovulation when looking forward to the next cycle. Its greatest utility is that it increases your awareness during the appropriate time in the cycle. In particular, couples who calculate the Average Day of Ovulation

(ADO) should be able to more accurately identify the time of ovulation by looking for other pieces of information such as Spinnbarkeit or Mittleschmerz at their most likely time of appearance.

Mittleschmerz/Bounce - this is considered merely a fair method of determining ovulation because it is only present in approximately 25% of women (Cunningham, 1993). In the fortunate minority of women who experience this pain regularly, it is an excellent predictor of ovulation. In fact, it should identify the time of ovulation more closely than BBT graphing, and it may be as accurate as cervical mucus determinations or urine LH determinations. The pain has been found to occur 24 to 48 hours prior to ovulation in the vast majority of women (O'Hearlihy et al, 1980). Intercourse can, therefore, begin 24 hours after the occurrence of the pain and continue for 48 to 72 hours or through the first day after the temperature rise.

The Bounce Test can elucidate ovulatory pain in up to one-third of women and, thus, should be attempted in any woman who does not appreciate the pain of Mittleschmerz.

Cervical Mucus Chemistry - this is considered only a fair method of determining ovulation because it relies on subjective assessment of the color presented on the glucose test paper which can be difficult. The key to determining ovulation is following the color change during successive cycles and identifying the peak color — the color with the darkest green or most blue — which corresponds roughly with the time of ovulation. Intercourse should occur in the next cycle when this color first appears.

Summary of Female Sex Preselection:

1. Read and study each method of ovulation detection discussed in the previous chapters.

2. Follow each method for three consecutive menstrual cycles and record all information on the Sex Preselection Charts. Use the following signs and symptoms, which have been arranged in order of decreasing accuracy and reliability, to identify the time of ovulation is each cycle:

   a. 16 to 28 hours after the first (+) LH determination
   b. 24 to 48 hours after Mittleschmerz/Bounce pain is felt
   c. The Peak Symptom is identified
   d. A high and soft cervix with a patent os is palpated
   e. Midway between the BBT nadir and the BBT rise
   f. glucose test paper reaches its darkest color
   g. The day of ovulation is estimated from the calendar

3. Analyze each chart and record the following lengths of time or days on the Cycle Summary Calculation Sheets:

   MCL - Menstrual Cycle Length
   DO - Day of Ovulation
   LPL - Luteal Phase Length

4. After the second cycle, the Cycle Summary Calculation Sheet should be used to calculate the Average Day of Ovulation (ADO).

5. At the beginning of the cycle during which preselection will take place, use a vertical line, labelled "O", on the BBT graph to mark the ADO on the upcoming Sex Preselection Chart. You should watch more closely for other indicators of ovulation as this day approaches.

6. Place a second vertical line, labelled "F", exactly six days prior to the ADO line. This represents the estimated beginning of the fertile period — the AFP. As this day approaches, watch closely for early cervical mucus production, concentrate on finding Mittleschmerz or Bounce pain, and begin to test urine samples for LH on at least a daily basis. Intercourse should cease at this time to avoid intercourse during a time which might result in more male children.

7. Approximately 48 hours before the ADO, examine the urine LH tests closely for a positive result. If not already taking place, urine should begin to be tested in both the morning and the evening. Also, women who experience Mittleschmerz or Bounce pain should be actively seeking the pain at this time.

8. After the first appearance of Mittleschmerz or Bounce pain, ovulation should occur in 24 to 48 hours. After the first positive LH result, discontinue urine testing: ovulation should occur in just less than 24 hours.

9. Within the above time periods, intercourse should take place when the following signs and symptoms aggregate to indicate ovulation:

    a. The Peak Symptom is identified.
    b. A high and soft cervix with a patent os is palpated.
    c. The BBT drops to form the BBT nadir and then increases
    d. glucose test paper reaches its darkest color.
    e. The ADO arrives.

Notice that, although this list has been constructed in order of decreasing accuracy and reliability, all of the methods can yield valuable information. We strongly recommend the use of **all** of the methods.

10. The identification of the basal body temperature shift generally indicates that ovulation has already occurred, and the days of higher male probability will soon begin. Thus, we recommend that intercourse cease shortly after the shift. If intercourse has not occurred and the shift is noted, we would recommend waiting until the next cycle to attempt preselection.

11. Intercourse can reasonably occur once at the estimated time of ovulation or more than once during the period 24 hours before to 24 hours after the estimated time.

12. Use the rear-entry position during intercourse — this will place the ejaculated semen very near to the opening of the cervix.

13. Immediately after insemination, the female partner should rest on her back with a pillow underneath her hips and remain still with her legs together for approximately 30 minutes; this will promote movement of sperm up the female tract.

14. When a child is conceived, compare the time of intercourse with the day of ovulation as determined after the cycle has ended. Then, consult the graphs in Chapter III to estimate the probability that the new child is a female.

15. If a child is not conceived after 12 cycles, we recommend consultation with your gynecologist or family physician. Female Sex Preselection should place intercourse at a time when the probability of conception is very high, and the absence of fertilization after 12 cycles is, by definition, infertility.

"Organizing is what you do before you do something, so that when you do it, it's not all mixed up."
A.A. Milne

Chapter XIII

Cycle Summary Calculation Sheet

This sheet has been provided to simplify the calculation of average values. All average values are calculated using the following formula:

$$\text{Average Value} = \frac{\text{Sum of All Recorded Values}}{\text{Total Number of Cycles}}$$

At the end of each cycle, record the following values on the chart:

MCL = Menstrual Cycle Length
LPL = Luteal Phase Length
DO = Day of Ovulation

Averages, by definition, cannot be calculated until at least two values are obtained. Thus, on the second and successive cycles, calculate the following averages:

$$\textbf{ACL} = \text{Average Cycle Length}$$
$$\textbf{ALPL} = \text{Average Luteal Phase Length}$$
$$\textbf{ADO} = \text{Average Day of Ovulation}$$

Finally, calculate the average day on which the fertile period begins:

$$\textbf{AFP} = \textbf{ADO - 6}$$

After all of the average values have been calculated, record them at the top of the next Sex Preselection Chart.

A double-sided CSCS can be found at the end of this book immediately after the bibliography; it has been perforated for easy removal. Additional copies may be obtained by contacting:

Young Ideas
1600 South Coulter Blvd.
Bldg C, Suite 304
Amarillo, Texas 79106

Chapter XIV

Sex Preselection Charts

We have discussed in detail the research on sex preselection and each method for determining ovulation at home. The information gained during close observation of the menstrual cycle will be very difficult to interpret unless it is put in to an organized form. To accomplish this, we have provided the Sex Preselection Charts at the end of this book; they are perforated and can be removed for easy use. In Chapters VI through X, we presented our recommendations on abbreviations which will easily fit into the spaces provided on the chart. In this chapter, we will examine each section of the chart and review our recommendations.

1. Chart Identification

Chart #:

In the upper left corner of the chart is the location in which the chart number should be recorded. Although it will be easy to identify the charts during the first few months, it may take many cycles of observation to become comfortable identifying the fertile period and ovulation. Numbered charts will make it easy to place them in the proper order.

Month and Day:

At the beginning of each cycle, the month and day should be recorded above the day of the cycle. Knowledge of the day of the month will help ensure that days are not skipped. In addition, the exact date will be important information for your obstetrician when the act of intercourse results in fertilization; this date can be used to predict the time at which the baby will be delivered.

2. Calendar Recording

This method can be used to look back at the cycle and identify ovulation; and, after a few cycles have been carefully examined, it can be used to predict the day of ovulation. When the cycle length is known, the luteal phase length (**LPL**) is subtracted from the cycle length (**MCL**) to find the proposed day of ovulation (**DO**):

$$\textbf{MCL} = \text{Menstrual Cycle Length}$$
$$\textbf{LPL} = \text{Luteal Phase Length}$$
$$\textbf{DO} = \text{Day of Ovulation}$$

$$\textbf{DO} = \textbf{MCL} - \textbf{LPL}$$

The above equations can be made more accurate by using the average lengths across all of the cycles charted. The previous chapter has all of the formulas to calculate:

$$\textbf{ACL} = \text{Average Cycle Length}$$
$$\textbf{ALPL} = \text{Average Luteal Phase Length}$$
$$\textbf{ADO} = \text{Average Day of Ovulation}$$

It should be noted that the ADO will become more useful as more cycles are used to find the average values. It will not, however, accurately predict ovulation in women with irregular cycles.

3. Basal Body Temperature Graphing

Accurate temperatures should be carefully graphed as a black dot under the day of the cycle. If any interfering factor can be identified, it should be described briefly by writing vertically under the day of the cycle. Temperatures higher than 99.0 F should be written at the top of the graph under the day of the cycle while those temperatures below 97.0 F should be written below the graph. Each new temperature dot should be connected by a line to the previous temperatures to produce the "temperature curve". Finally, intercourse should be designated by placing a star (*) over the temperature — again, this knowledge will become very important after fertilization has occurred.

4. Cervical Mucus Changes

The chart has four spaces under each day of the menstrual cycle to describe the cervical mucus properties designated quantity, consistency, and translucency. We suggest the following descriptive terms.

QUANTITY:
- **D** = none or dry
- **S** = slight
- **M** = moderate
- **A** = abundant

CONSISTENCY:
T = thick
ST = sticky
M = moderate
SL = slippery
W = watery

TRANSLUCENCY:
O = opaque
C = cloudy
T = translucent or clear

If the presence of a Peak Symptom or Spinnbarkeit is noted, **PS** or **SBK** should be written in the fourth row labelled Signs.

5. Cervical Changes

Under each day of the cycle, locations have been reserved for charting the os diameter, texture, and position of the cervix. Each location is only large enough to accommodate one letter. Therefore, we suggest the following designations:

Os Diameter:
S = Small
I = Intermediate
L = Large

Texture:
F = Firm
I = Intermediate
S = Soft

Position:
L = Low
I = Intermediate
H = High

6. Mittleschmerz / Bounce

The presence of Mittleschmerz or bounce pain should be graphed under the day of its occurrence. There is room for only a single letter designation and we recommend:

$$\begin{aligned} \mathbf{M} &= \text{Mittleschmerz} \\ \mathbf{B} &= \text{Bounce} \end{aligned}$$

Place a 0 in the box if this pain was watched for closely but not noted or if the Bounce Test was performed without pain elicited.

7. Cervical Mucus Chemistry

Changes noted in the color of glucose test paper should be graphed under the appropriate day of the cycle. We recommend the following designations:

Color Chart Method:
$$\begin{aligned} 0 &= 0 \\ 1 &= + \\ 2 &= ++ \\ 3 &= +++ \\ 4 &= ++++ \end{aligned}$$

Descriptive Method:
$$\begin{aligned} \mathbf{Y} &= \text{Yellow} \\ \mathbf{YG} &= \text{Yellow - Green} \\ \mathbf{G} &= \text{Green} \\ \mathbf{BG} &= \text{Blue - Green} \\ \mathbf{B} &= \text{Blue — possible ovulation} \\ \mathbf{DB} &= \text{Dark Blue — indicative of ovulation} \end{aligned}$$

8. Urine LH Determinations

Each result from a urinary LH determination should be graphed with a (-) or (+) under the appropriate day of the cycle. Morning results are graphed above the slash (/) while evening results are graphed below it. After the first positive test there is no reason to test for further LH in the urine.

9. Additional Information

Space has been set aside at the bottom of each chart to allow you to graph any additional information which helps you to identify the time of ovulation with more accuracy. Careful observation during each menstrual cycle in a particular woman may reveal other indicators of the time of ovulation. <u>We hope that you will use this section to individualize the process of sex preselection.</u>

"It is a bad plan that admits of no modification."
Publilius Syrus

Double-sided Female Sex Preselection Charts can be found at the end of this book, immediately after the Cycle Summary Calculation Sheets; they have been perforated for easy removal. Additional copies may be obtained by contacting:

Young Ideas
1600 South Coulter Blvd.
Bldg. C, Suite 304
Amarillo, Texas 79106
(806) 353-8436

GLOSSARY

Acidic - the term used to describe a substance which liberates hydrogen ions into solution; these substances have a pH from 0 to just less than 7; examples of acidic substances include vinegar and the secretions of the stomach and the vagina.

ACL see Average Cycle Length

ADO see Average Day of Ovulation

AFP see Average First Day of the Fertile Period

ALPL see Average Luteal Phase Length

Androsperm - the term used by Dr. Shettles to describe sperm bearing the Y sex chromosome; fertilization by such sperm will result in male offspring.

Artificial insemination - the placement of sperm into the female reproductive tract by artificial means — not by direct discharge from a penis; homologous artificial insemination describes the placement of sperm obtained from the mate of the female while heterologous artificial insemination describes the placement of sperm obtained from other than the mate.

Average Cycle Length - the average length of the menstrual cycles of a given female which is found by adding the lengths of each cycle and dividing by the total number of cycles.

Average Day of Ovulation - the average day of ovulation of a given female which is found by adding the number of days in each cycle prior to ovulation and dividing by the number of cycles examined.

Average First Day of the Fertile Period - that day, abbreviated **AFP**, which is 6 days prior to the Average Day of Ovulation (ADO) calculated as follows:
$$AFP = ADO - 6$$

Average Luteal Phase Length - the average length of the luteal phase of a given female which is found by adding the lengths of each luteal phase and dividing by the total number of phases.

Basal Body Temperature - the temperature of the body at rest, without the interference of activity which tends to increase the body temperature; this temperature is, therefore, more influenced by the hormonal state of the body and is optimal for indicating the phase of the menstrual cycle in ovulating females.

Basal Body Temperature nadir - a drop in the basal body temperature which may precede the progesterone induced BBT rise near ovulation; for the purpose of sex preselection, we will consider a BBT nadir to occur 0.5 days prior to ovulation.

Basal Body Temperature shift - the increase in basal body temperature which occurs within 48 hours of ovulation in the majority of women; for the purposes of sex preselection, we will consider ovulation to occur 0.5 days prior to this BBT shift.

Basic - the term used to describe a substance which combines with hydrogen ions; these substances have a pH from just greater than 7 to 14; examples of basic substances include baking soda, lye, and semen.

BBT see Basal Body Temperature

BBT Nadir see Basal Body Temperature Nadir

Bounce test - a test introduced by Dr. H. Shapiro in 1978 which may help to define the time of ovulation by augmenting the pain of Mittleschmerz — the woman is instructed to move abruptly to a sitting position three to four times a day beginning six days prior to the expected time of ovulation; sharp pains in the lower abdomen during such position changes have been associated with ovulation in a small number of women.

Boy days - those days in which the probability of conceiving a male child is greater; in our method, this would correspond to those days which are 4 or more days prior to ovulation.

Calendar method - a marginally effective method of birth control in which the time of fertility or ovulation is estimated based on examination of previous menstrual cycles; ovulation is predicted to occur 14 days (12 to 16) prior to the expected end of the menstrual cycle — this method is more successful in the minority of women with regular menstrual cycle lengths.

Cervical mucus - mucus produced by glands in the cervical canal; cervical glands are responsive to changes in circulating female hormones, and changes in cervical mucus can indicate the time of ovulation.

Cervix - the lower one-third of the uterus which lies between the body of the uterus and the vaginal canal

Chadwick's sign - the enlargement, softening, and bluish discoloration often noted in the cervix of a pregnant female due to the marked increase in blood flow.

Chromosome - a structure found in the nucleus of a cell which contains and transmits genetic information; each human somatic (non-sex) cell contains 23 pairs of chromosomes including one pair of sex chromosomes, XX in a female or XY in a male.

Corpus luteum - the cells of the ovarian follicle after ovulation which form a small yellow body that secretes increased amounts of progesterone.

Day of ovulation - the day upon which ovulation is thought to occur as indicated by basal body temperature graphing, mucus determinations, urinary LH monitoring, etc.

DO see Day of Ovulation

Douche, vaginal - the directed flow of fluid into the vagina in order to cleanse, treat infection, deodorize, or alter the pH; this is unnecessary in the normal, healthy female, can predispose to infection, and is not felt to be effective as a method of contraception.

Egg - the female sex cell which contains one-half of the number of chromosomes found in a non-sex (somatic) cell — each egg has one X chromosome.

Estrogen - the hormone secreted by the ovaries in response to follicle stimulating hormone (FSH) secreted by the pituitary gland of the brain; it is responsible for the sex characteristics associated with females and for the maintenance of the female reproductive tract.

Fallopian tubes - the portion of the female reproductive tract which lies between the uterus and the ovaries on each side; they transmit the egg to the uterus and are a common site of both fertilization and ectopic gestations; they are also known as oviducts.

Female reproductive tract - the organs of female reproduction including the ovaries, fallopian tubes, uterus, cervix, and vagina.

Fertile period - that period of time during which intercourse can with reasonable probability result in fertilization; we consider this period to consist of 8 days including 6 days prior to ovulation and 2 days after ovulation.

Fertilization - the union of a sperm and egg to form a zygote which usually occurs in the fallopian tubes.

Fimbria - finger-like projections located at the end of each fallopian tube next to or touching the ovaries which help to guide the ovulated egg into the tube.

First Day of the Fertile Period - that day, abbreviated FP, which is 6 days prior to the Day of Ovulation (DO) calculated as follows:

$$FP = DO - 6$$

Follicle stimulating hormone - the hormone secreted by the pituitary gland of the brain which stimulates the maturation of the ovarian follicle and production of estrogen in females.

Follicular phase - the term used to describe the time during the menstrual cycle after menstruation and prior to ovulation during which the follicular cells secrete high quantities of estrogen.

FP see First Day of the Fertile Period

FSH see Follicle Stimulating Hormone

Girl days - those days upon which the probability of conceiving a female child is greatest; in our method, this would correspond to the 3 day period which includes the day before, the day of, and the day after ovulation.

Guaifenesin - an agent which dissolves mucus (mucolytic); it is found in many of the over-the-counter cold and sinus medications.

Gynosperm - the term used by Dr. Shettles to describe sperm bearing an X sex chromosome; fertilization by such sperm will result in female offspring.

Hormone - a substance produced in one area of the body which is carried by the blood to another area of the body upon which it has an effect.

Ideal cycle - the term used to describe a 28 day menstrual cycle in which ovulation occurs near day 14.

LH see Luteinizing Hormone

LPL see Luteal Phase Length

Luteal Phase - the term used to describe the time during the menstrual cycle after ovulation and prior to the next menstruation during which the corpus luteum secretes increasing quantities of progesterone.

Luteal phase length - the length in days of the luteal phase.

Luteinizing Hormone - the hormone secreted by the pituitary gland of the brain in response to increased estrogen levels in females which induces ovulation and the formation of the corpus luteum which secretes progesterone.

MCL see Menstrual Cycle Length

Menstrual cycle - the designation for one complete series of cyclic changes in the female reproductive tract beginning with menstruation and ending just prior to the next menstruation; each menstrual cycle includes menstruation, a follicular phase, ovulation, and a luteal phase.

Menstrual Cycle Length - the length in days of the menstrual cycle.

Menstruation - the periodic sloughing of the uterine inner lining as a bloody discharge occurring regularly from menarche to menopause at the beginning of each menstrual cycle.

Midcycle - the middle of a menstrual cycle; it is designed to refer to ovulation since, in the ideal 28 day cycle, ovulation occurs on day 14 - the middle of the cycle.

Mittleschmerz - a sharp abdominal pain that occurs shortly before the time of ovulation in a small number (approximately 25%) of women.

Mucus - the thick and slippery secretion of mucous membranes and glands such as those of the cervix; it serves to moisten and protect them and is composed of a protein called mucin, water, salts, and cells of the body.

Os - the term used to describe an opening; we use it to describe the opening of the cervix as entered from the vagina.

Ovulation - the rupture of a mature ovarian follicle with release of an egg which occurs near the middle of the menstrual cycle.

Peak symptom - see Spinnbarkeit

Progesterone - the female hormone which is produced primarily after ovulation and acts to prepare the uterus for implantation of a fertilized egg; it is produced initially by the corpus luteum and later by the placenta.

Rhythm method - a method of contraception which uses calendar charting, basal body temperature charting, and examination of mucus changes to determine the fertile period.

Sex chromosomes - the two chromosomes in each somatic (non-sex) cell, XX in females and XY in males, which determine the sexual characteristics of the individual; each egg of a female contain only one X chromosome while each sperm of a male contains either one X or one Y chromosome.

Sex preselection - the ability to influence the sex of offspring prior to birth.

Speculum, vaginal - an instrument used by physicians to view the vagina and cervix.

Spinnbarkeit - the term used to describe the elastic quality of cervical mucus at the time of ovulation.

Statistical significance - the designation that an occurrence has been analyzed statistically and found to have had only a small percentage chance (usually less than 5% chance) of having occurred randomly.

Temperature curve - the term for the curve formed when basal body temperatures are graphed against the days of the menstrual cycle.

Tes-Tape® - a strip of paper impregnated with chemicals which react with glucose and cause the color of the paper to change; it is produced by Eli Lilly and Company and may be used to identify the time of ovulation.

X chromosome - the chromosome that determines the characteristics of the female sex; one of the two types of sex chromosomes, X and Y.

X sperm - sperm which contain the X chromosome and result in the conception of female offspring; synonymous with gynosperm.

Y chromosome - the chromosome that determines the characteristics of the male sex; one of the two types of sex chromosomes, X and Y.

Y sperm - sperm which contain the Y chromosome and result in the conception of male offspring; synonymous with androsperm.

BIBLIOGRAPHY

"A man will turn over half a library to make one book."
Johnson

Abrams RM, Royston JP: Some properties of rectum and vagina as sites for basal body temperature measurement. *Fertil Steril* 35:313, 1981.

Bartzen PJ: Effectiveness of the temperature rhythm system of contraception. *Fertil Steril* 18:694, 1967.

Billings EL, Billings JJ, Brown JB, Burger HG: Symptoms and hormonal changes accompanying ovulation. *Lancet,* Feb 5, 1972.

Birnberg CH, Kurzrok R, Laufer A: Simple test for determining ovulation time. *JAMA* 166:1174, 1958.

Cunningham FG, et al: ***William's Obstetrics***. Appleton and Lange, Norwalk, Conn., 1993.

Duffy, MA: ***Physicians' Desk Reference, 46th Edition***. Medical Economics Data, Montvale, NJ, 1992.

France JT, Graham FM, Gosling L, Hair FI: A prospective study of the preselection of the sex of offspring by timing intercourse relative to ovulation. *Fert Steril* 41:894-900, 1984.

Grinsted J, Jacobsen JD, Grinsted L, Schantz A, Stenfoss HH, Nielson SP: Prediction of ovulation. *Fert Steril* 32(3):388-393, 1989.

Guerrero RV: Association of the type and time of insemination within the menstrual cycle with the human sex ratio at birth. *N Engl J Med* 291:1056-1059, 1974.

Guerrero RV, Rojas, OI: Spontaneous abortion and aging of human ova and spermatozoa. *N Engl J Med* 293(12):573-575, 1975.

Guttmacher AF: Factors affecting normal expectancy of conception. *JAMA* 161:855, 1956.

Harlap S: Gender of infants conceived on different days of the menstrual cycle. *N Engl J Med* 300:1445-1448, 1979.

Hilgers TW, Abraham GE, Cavanaugh D: Natural family planning. I. The peak symptom and estimated time of ovulation. *Obstet Gynecol* 52(5):575-582, 1978.

Hilgers TW, Bailey AJ: Natural family planning. II. Basal body temperature and estimated time of ovulation. *Obstet Gynecol* 55:333, 1980.

Lampe KF: *American Medical Association Drug Evaluations, 6th Edition.* Chicago, IL, 1986.

Luciano AA, Peluso J, Koch EI, Maier D, Kuslis S, Davison E: Temporal relationship and reliability of the clinical, hormonal, and ultrasonographic indices of ovulation in infertile women. *Obstet Gynecol* 75:412, 1990.

Marinho AO, Sallam HN, Goessens LKV, Collins WP, Rodeck CH, Campbell S: Real time pelvic ultrasonography during the periovulatory period of patients attending an artificial insemination clinic. *Fertil Steril* 37:633, 1982.

Martinez AR, Bernardus RE, Kucharska D, Schoemaker J: Urinary luteinizing hormone testing and prediction of ovulation in spontaneous, clomiphene citrate and human menopausal gonadotropin-stimulated cycles. A clinical evaluation. *Acta Endrocrinologica* 124:357-363, 1991.

Moghissi KS: Prediction and detection of ovulation. *Fertil Steril* 34:89, 1980.

O'Herlihy C, Robinson HP, Crespigny LJChDe: Mittleschmerz is a preovulatory symptom. *Br Med J* 280:986, 1980.

Perez A, Eger R, Domenichini V: Sex Ratio Associated with Natural Family Planning. *Fertil Steril* 43:152-153, 1985.

Royston JP: Basal body temperature, ovulation and the risk of conception, with special reference to the lifetimes of sperm and egg. *Biometrics* 38:397-406, 1982.

Seikel MM, Shine W, Smith DM: Biological rhythm of the lutenizing hormone surge. *Fertil Steril* 37:709-711, 1982.

Shapiro HI: *The Birth Control Book*. Avon Books, 1978.

Shettles LB: Factors influencing sex ratios. *Int J Gynecol Obstet* 8:643, 1970.

Shettles LB, Rorvik DM: *Your Baby's Sex: now you can choose.* Dodd, Mead and Company, 1970.

Simcock BW: Sons and Daughters — a sex preselection study. *Med J Aust* 142:541, 1985.

Singh M, Saxena BB, Rathnam P: Clinical valication of enzyme immunoassay of human luteinizing hormone (hLH) in the detection of the preovulatory luteinizing hormone (LH) surge in urine. *Fertil Steril* 41:210-217, 1984.

Testart J, Thebault A, Souderes E, Frydman R: Premature ovulation after ovarian ultrasonography. *Br J Obstet Gynaecol* 89:694, 1982.

Thomas CL: *Taber's Cyclopedic Medical Dictionary*. F. A. Davis Company, 1981.

Vermesh M, Kletzky OA, Val Davajan IR: Monitoring techniques to predict and detect ovulation. *Fertil Steril* 47:259-264, 1987.

World Health Organization: A prospective multicenter study of the ovulation method of natural family planning. IV. The outcome of pregnancy. *Fertil Steril* 41:593-598, 1984.

Zarutskie PW, Muller CH, Magone M, Soules MR: The clinical relevance of sex selection techniques. *Fertil Steril* 52(6):891-905, 1989.

Zuspan KJ, Zuspan FP: Thermogenic alterations in the woman. *Am J Obstet Gynecol* 120:441, 1974.

"The writer does the most who gives his reader the most knowledge and takes from him the least time."

Sydney Smith

"In this work, when it shall be found that much is omitted, let it not be forgotten that much likewise is performed." — **Dr. Samuel Johnson** upon completion of his dictionary, 1755.

Order Form

Telephone Orders: Call Toll Free

1-800-213-BABY

Have your Mastercard or Visa ready.

Fax Orders: (806) 354-2810

Postal Orders: Young Ideas, Publishing Division
1600 South Coulter, Bldg C, Suite 304
Amarillo, Texas 79106

**Please send me the following books or materials. I understand that I may
promptly return any unused books or materials for a full refund.**

Company Name: _____

Name: _____

Address: _____

City: _____ State: _____ Zip: _____-_____

How To Have A Boy	$19.95 ea.	Qty. _____
12 Male Charts (8.5 x 11)	$3.00 ea. set	Qty. _____
How To Have A Girl	$19.95 ea.	Qty. _____
12 Female Charts (8.5 x 11)	$3.00 ea. set	Qty. _____

Please add 8.25% Sales Tax for books shipped to Texas addresses.

Shipping and Handling:
 ☐ Air Mail: $4.00 per book
 ☐ Book Rate: $2.00 for the first book
                       $1.00 for each additional book

                       Please allow 4 to 6 weeks for delivery

Payment:
 ☐ Check
 ☐ Credit Card: Visa   Mastercard

            Card Number: _____

            Name on Card: _____

            Expiration Date: _____ / _____

Order Now ... Toll Free

Cycle Summary Calculation Sheet

Cycle #	MCL	DO	LPL	ACL	ADO	ALPL
1						
2						
3						
4						
5						
6						
7						
8						
9						
10						
11						
12						

Cycle Summary Calculation Sheet

Cycle #	MCL	DO	LPL	ACL	ADO	ALPL
1						
2						
3						
4						
5						
6						
7						
8						
9						
10						
11						
12						

Chart # —

Female Sex Preselection Chart

CSCS Information	Present Cycle Valves

CSCS Information

ACL = Average Cycle Length = ————
ALPL = Average Luteal Phase Length = ————
ADO = Average Day of Ovulation = ————

Present Cycle Valves

MCL = Menstrual Cycle Length = ————
LPL = Luteal Phase Length = ————
DO = Day of Ovulation = ————

Day of the Month																																							
Month																																							
Day of the Cycle	1	2	3	4	5	6	7	8	9	10	11	12	13	14	15	16	17	18	19	20	21	22	23	24	25	26	27	28	29	30	31	32	33	34	35	36	37	38	39	40

Basal Body Temperature (99.0, .8, .6, .4, .2, 98.0, .8, .6, .4, .2, 97.0)

Mucus: Quantity, Consistency, Translucency

Signs

Cervix: Os Diameter, Texture, Position

Mittleschmerz/Bounce
Glucose/TesTape
Urine LH Tests

Non Specific Symptoms

Chart # ___

Female Sex Preselection Chart

CSCS Information		Present Cycle Valves	
ACL = Average Cycle Length = _____		MCL = Menstrual Cycle Length = _____	
ALPL = Average Luteal Phase Length = _____		LPL = Luteal Phase Length= _____	
ADO = Average Day of Ovulation = _____		DO = Day of Ovulation = _____	

	Day of the Month																																								
	Month																																								
	Day of the Cycle	1	2	3	4	5	6	7	8	9	10	11	12	13	14	15	16	17	18	19	20	21	22	23	24	25	26	27	28	29	30	31	32	33	34	35	36	37	38	39	40
Basal Body Temperature	99.0 .8 .6 .4 .2 98.0 .8 .6 .4 .2 97.0																																								
Mucus	Quantity																																								
	Consistency																																								
	Translucency																																								
	Signs																																								
Cervix	Os Diameter																																								
	Texture																																								
	Position																																								
Mittleschmerz/Bounce																																										
Glucose/TesTape																																										
Urine LH Tests																																										
Non Specific Symptoms																																										

Chart # ____

Female Sex Preselection Chart

CSCS Information

ACL = Average Cycle Length = _____

ALPL = Average Luteal Phase Length = _____

ADO = Average Day of Ovulation = _____

Present Cycle Valves

MCL = Menstrual Cycle Length = _____

LPL = Luteal Phase Length= _____

DO = Day of Ovulation = _____

Day of the Month																																							
Month																																							
Day of the Cycle	1	2	3	4	5	6	7	8	9	10	11	12	13	14	15	16	17	18	19	20	21	22	23	24	25	26	27	28	29	30	31	32	33	34	35	36	37	38	39	40

Basal Body Temperature — 99.0, .8, .6, .4, .2, 98.0, .8, .6, .4, .2, 97.0

Mucus
- Quantity
- Consistency
- Translucency

Cervix
- Signs
- Os Diameter
- Texture
- Position

- Mittelschmerz/Bounce
- Glucose/TesTape
- Urine LH Tests

- Non Specific Symptoms

Female Sex Preselection Chart

Chart # ___

CSCS Information

	Present Cycle Valves	
ACL = Average Cycle Length = ___	MCL = Menstrual Cycle Length = ___	
ALPL = Average Luteal Phase Length = ___	LPL = Luteal Phase Length= ___	
ADO = Average Day of Ovulation = ___	DO = Day of Ovulation = ___	

	Day of the Month																																							
	Month																																							
	Day of the Cycle	1	2	3	4	5	6	7	8	9	10	11	12	13	14	15	16	17	18	19	20	21	22	23	24	25	26	27	28	29	30	31	32	33	34	35	36	37	38	39	40
Basal Body Temperature	99.0 .8 .6 .4 .2 98.0 .8 .6 .4 .2 97.0																																								
Mucus	Quantity																																								
	Consistency																																								
	Translucency																																								
Cervix	Signs																																								
	Os Diameter																																								
	Texture																																								
	Position																																								
	Mittleschmerz/Bounce																																								
	Glucose/TesTape																																								
	Urine LH Tests																																								
	Non Specific Symptoms																																								

Female Sex Preselection Chart

Chart # —

CSCS Information

ACL = Average Cycle Length = _____

ALPL = Average Luteal Phase Length = _____

ADO = Average Day of Ovulation = _____

Present Cycle Valves

MCL = Menstrual Cycle Length = _____

LPL = Luteal Phase Length = _____

DO = Day of Ovulation = _____

Day of the Month																																								
Month																																								
Day of the Cycle	1	2	3	4	5	6	7	8	9	10	11	12	13	14	15	16	17	18	19	20	21	22	23	24	25	26	27	28	29	30	31	32	33	34	35	36	37	38	39	40

Basal Body Temperature: 99.0, .8, .6, .4, .2, 98.0, .8, .6, .4, .2, 97.0

Mucus: Quantity, Consistency, Translucency

Signs

Cervix: Os Diameter, Texture, Position

Mittleschmerz/Bounce

Glucose/TesTape

Urine LH Tests

Non Specific Symptoms

Female Sex Preselection Chart

Chart # ___

CSCS Information	Present Cycle Valves

ACL. = Average Cycle Length = _____

ALPL = Average Luteal Phase Length = _____

ADO = Average Day of Ovulation = _____

MCL. = Menstrual Cycle Length = _____

LPL = Luteal Phase Length = _____

DO = Day of Ovulation = _____

		Day of the Month																																								
		Month																																								
		Day of the Cycle	1	2	3	4	5	6	7	8	9	10	11	12	13	14	15	16	17	18	19	20	21	22	23	24	25	26	27	28	29	30	31	32	33	34	35	36	37	38	39	40
Basal Body Temperature	99.0 .8 .6 .4 .2 98.0 .8 .6 .4 .2 97.0																																									
Mucus	Quantity																																										
	Consistency																																										
	Translucency																																										
Cervix	Signs																																										
	Texture																																										
	Os Diameter																																										
	Position																																										
Mintleschmerz/Bounce																																											
Glucose/TesTape																																											
Urine LH Tests																																											
Non Specific Symptoms																																											